PALEO SLOW COOKER

**75 Easy, Healthy, and Delicious Gluten-Free
Paleo Slow Cooker Recipes for a Paleo Diet**

By John Chatham

ROCKRIDGE
UNIVERSITY PRESS

CONTENTS

Chapter 3: Soups, Stews, and Stocks

Contents

Chapter 4: Meat Entrées

Contents

INTRODUCTION

Paleo cooking and the slow cooker go beautifully together. Because the Paleo and gluten-free diets are focused on whole foods, it can be time-intensive to prepare meals, especially on busy weeknights. A slow cooker makes it possible to cook wonderful meals from healthful, whole foods with far less time—and it can also politely have dinner waiting for you when you get home.

Cooking your meals in a slow cooker can also make the Paleo and gluten-free diet easier on the budget. Slow cooking makes it possible to creatively turn a budget cut of meat into a succulent, tender dish. Because the cooking takes place at a steady, slow temperature, flavors and juices are sealed in, and wonderful sauces and gravies can be made from the cooking liquids.

Slow cooking also helps you to keep all of the vitamins, minerals, and antioxidants present in your foods from being lost, as they would during many other cooking methods. This means your meals are not only delicious, they're also much better for you.

Most important, if you've been hesitant to start your Paleo and gluten-free diet because you think you just don't have the time to do all of the cooking, your slow cooker can help you make that healthful decision and stick to it.

Collected here are some of the most delicious and easy-to-prepare Paleo and gluten-free slow cooker recipes, and everything you need to know to use your slow cooker successfully. Now there's no reason why you can't start your Paleo and gluten-free diet right away, or for your current Paleo menu to rely on only a few tried-and-true dishes.

Paleo and Gluten-Free Slow Cooker Recipes

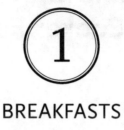

BREAKFASTS

Steamed Hazelnut Breakfast Bread

This recipe is a bit like a lighter version of steamed brown bread. The hazelnut flour, walnuts, and almond milk give it a deliciously nutty flavor with a hint of sweetness. It's perfect for breakfast or a snack.

- 1 to 1 1/2 cups hot water
- 1 1/2 cups hazelnut flour
- 1 teaspoon baking soda
- 1/2 teaspoon ground cinnamon
- 1/2 teaspoon ground nutmeg
- 1/2 teaspoon sea salt
- 1 cup unflavored almond milk
- 1/3 cup raw honey
- 1/2 cup chopped walnuts
- 1 teaspoon walnut oil

Turn the slow cooker on low heat and pour in enough hot water to reach a depth of about 1 inch. Place a cake or grilling rack in the slow cooker or use 4 fist-sized balls of aluminum foil as a homemade rack. Place the lid on the slow cooker.

In a large mixing bowl, combine the hazelnut flour, baking soda, cinnamon, nutmeg, and salt, and mix with a wooden spoon or whisk until well blended. Add the almond milk and honey, and mix just until fully combined. Do not overmix. Fold in the walnuts and stir until incorporated.

Grease a 2-quart soufflé dish or deep casserole with the walnut oil and pour in the batter, spreading it evenly. Cover with foil and place the dish on the rack in the slow cooker.

Cover and cook on low heat for 3 hours, or until a toothpick inserted into the center of the bread comes out clean. Carefully remove both the dish and rack, remove the foil, and cool the dish on the rack for 10 to 15 minutes before loosening the edges of the bread with a knife. Transfer the bread to the rack to cool for another 10 minutes before slicing.

Serves 8.

Poached Pears with Cranberries

Sometimes you just want something sweet alongside your Paleo-friendly omelet. These poached pears fit the bill nicely, and they reheat well if you'd like to make a large batch to eat during the week.

- 8 firm pears, such as Bosc, peeled and cored
- 1/2 teaspoon ground cinnamon
- 1/2 teaspoon ground nutmeg
- 2 tablespoons coconut oil
- 1/2 cup raw honey
- 1/2 teaspoon pure vanilla extract
- 1 cup dried unsweetened cranberries

Slice a very thin slice from the bottom of each pear to help the fruit stand upright.

In a small dish or bowl, combine the cinnamon and nutmeg, and sprinkle over the pears. Place the pears upright in the slow cooker.

Combine the coconut oil and honey in a small saucepan. Warm over low heat just until melted. Remove from heat and stir in the vanilla. Pour the mixture over the pears, then add cranberries to the slow cooker, distributing them evenly around the pears.

Cover and cook on low heat for 4 hours. To serve, place a pear on a small plate, spoon cranberries around it, and drizzle a little of the cooking liquid over the top.

Serves 8.

Dried Berry Compote

This easy compote makes a great topping for Paleo pancakes or waffles on weekend mornings. It keeps well in the fridge for about a week in a tightly covered jar or dish.

- 1/2 cup raw honey
- 1/2 teaspoon pure vanilla extract
- 1/2 teaspoon pure almond extract
- 1/2 teaspoon ground cinnamon
- 1/2 teaspoon ground cloves
- 1 cup dried unsweetened Bing cherries
- 1/2 cup dried unsweetened blueberries
- 1/2 cup dried unsweetened cranberries

In a medium saucepan over low heat, combine the honey, vanilla and almond extracts, cinnamon, and cloves. Cook until the honey is just melted, stirring frequently.

Stir in the cherries and berries until well coated, and pour the mixture into the slow cooker. Cover and cook on low heat for 8 hours or overnight. Serve warm over pancakes or waffles or as a side dish.

Serves 6.

Cuban Pork and Plantain Ropa-Style Hash

Ropa vieja is a popular Cuban classic made of shredded beef or pork. In Cuban restaurants, it's most often served as a lunch or dinner entrée, but in homes, it also doubles as a filling breakfast meal with scrambled eggs.

- 1 teaspoon ground cumin
- 1 teaspoon garlic powder
- 1 teaspoon sea salt
- 1/2 teaspoon freshly ground black pepper
- 1 (1 1/2-pound) pork sirloin roast, trimmed of visible fat
- 1 teaspoon olive oil
- 1/2 cup beef broth
- 1 bay leaf
- 4 plantains, peeled and cut in half

Combine the cumin, garlic powder, salt, and pepper in a small bowl, and rub all over the roast, coating it evenly.

In a large, heavy skillet, heat the olive oil over medium-high heat. Brown the roast on all sides, 3 to 4 minutes per side. Set the skillet aside.

Place the roast in the slow cooker, and add the beef broth and bay leaf. Cover and cook on low heat for 8 hours.

Meanwhile, brown the plantains in the skillet over medium-high heat, using the leftover juices from the roast. Set aside.

After the pork has cooked for 4 hours, add the plantains to the slow cooker, arranging them around the roast. Continue cooking for 4 more hours.

Transfer the roast to a cutting board to cool until it can be handled comfortably. While it cools, dice the plantains and set aside in a large bowl, making sure to remove the bay leaf.

Use clean hands or 2 forks to shred the pork, and combine with the plantains. To serve, ladle over or serve alongside scrambled eggs.

Serves 6.

Slow Cooker Pumpkin Butter

Pumpkin and apple butters are great ways to add a bit of sweetness to the Paleo diet. They're extremely easy to make in the slow cooker and are delicious served warm after cooking overnight. The pumpkin butter keeps well in the fridge for about a week in a tightly covered jar.

- 2 (15-ounce) cans pumpkin puree (not pie filling)
- 1/2 cup unsweetened apple juice
- 1/2 cup raw honey
- 1/2 teaspoon ground allspice
- 1/2 teaspoon ground nutmeg
- 1/2 teaspoon ground ginger
- 1/2 teaspoon sea salt

In a medium-sized bowl, combine the pumpkin puree, apple juice, and honey, and stir until well blended. Add the allspice, nutmeg, ginger, and salt, and stir well.

Pour the mixture into the slow cooker, cover, and cook on low heat for 8 hours. If the butter is a bit thin, uncover and increase the temperature to high heat. Allow the butter to reduce for about 30 minutes.

To serve, spread over Paleo-friendly breads, pancakes, or waffles, or use as a dip for fresh apple or pear slices.

Serves 12.

Vegetable Frittata

Frittatas are easily made Paleo friendly. Though they're also quick to make using traditional methods, having one ready and waiting in the slow cooker when you wake up is always nice.

- 12 large eggs, beaten
- 1/2 cup unflavored almond milk
- 1/2 cup diced red bell pepper
- 1/2 cup diced green bell pepper
- 1 medium white onion, diced
- 1 cup sliced white mushrooms
- 1 teaspoon sea salt
- 1/2 teaspoon freshly ground black pepper
- 1/2 teaspoon ground cumin
- 1 tablespoon olive oil

In a medium bowl, whisk the eggs and almond milk until well blended. Add the peppers, onion, and mushrooms. Mix well. Stir in the salt, pepper, and cumin.

Grease the bottom and halfway up the sides of the slow cooker crock with the olive oil. Pour in the egg mixture, cover, and cook on low heat for 8 hours. Serve warm with fresh fruit or Paleo-friendly muffins.

Serves 6.

Sweet Potato and Chicken-Sausage Hash

Commercial-cured sausage is off-limits to most Paleo followers, but there are several organic sausage brands that are fresh rather than cured and, therefore, perfectly acceptable. This recipe uses chicken sausage, which is one of the easier types to find.

- 1 pound chicken sausage, casing removed
- 4 large sweet potatoes, peeled and grated
- 2 firm apples, peeled, cored, and chopped
- 1 small white onion, diced
- 1/4 cup chicken broth or stock

In a large bowl, crumble the chicken sausage and combine with the sweet potatoes. Stir in the apples and onion, and press the mixture into the bottom of the slow cooker. Pour the broth over the top, cover, and cook on low heat for 8 hours or on high for 4 hours. Serve alongside eggs or on its own.

Serves 6.

SNACKS AND APPETIZERS

Slow Cooker Stuffed Portobellos

Stuffed mushrooms are a great appetizer to serve to company, and they also make an excellent light lunch or side dish for yourself. Portobellos are wonderfully dense—similar to steak—and delicious.

- 8 large portobello mushrooms
- 1 teaspoon olive oil
- 2 cloves garlic, crushed
- 1 teaspoon sea salt, divided
- 1/4 teaspoon freshly ground black pepper, divided
- 1/2 cup chopped pecans
- 1/2 cup diced white onion
- 1/2 cup frozen chopped spinach, thawed and drained well

Remove the stems from the mushrooms and chop them; set aside.

In a heavy skillet, heat the olive oil over medium heat. Add the garlic, 1/2 teaspoon salt, 1/8 teaspoon pepper, and pecans. Cook, stirring often, for about 5 minutes.

Add the onion, chopped mushroom stems, and spinach, stirring well, and cook for 1 minute to coat the pecans and vegetables with oil.

Use the remaining 1/2 teaspoon salt and 1/8 teaspoon pepper to season the mushroom caps.

Divide the mixture between the mushroom caps, spooning it loosely into each 1. Place the mushrooms in a single layer in the slow cooker. (It's okay if they are a bit crowded.) Cover and cook on low heat for 2 hours.

Serve as an appetizer or alongside a green salad for a light lunch.

Serves 4.

Spicy Slow Cooker–Roasted Nuts

Most people don't think to use slow cookers when it comes to preparing crunchy snacks, but it's actually a great no-fuss way to prepare tasty lunch-bag or party snacks for later. They're much lower in salt than commercially roasted nuts, too.

- 2 tablespoons olive oil
- 2 teaspoons garlic powder
- 1 teaspoon cayenne pepper
- 1 teaspoon onion powder
- 1 teaspoon paprika
- 1/2 teaspoon sea salt
- 1/2 pound pecan halves
- 1/2 pound walnut halves
- 1/2 pound shelled Brazil nuts

In a large bowl, combine the olive oil, garlic powder, cayenne pepper, onion powder, paprika, and salt, stirring until thoroughly blended. Add the pecans, walnuts, and Brazil nuts, and toss until the nuts are evenly coated.

Pour the nuts into the slow cooker and cover. Cook on high heat for 15 minutes. Toss again with a large spoon, cover, and cook on low for 2 hours.

Using a slotted spoon, transfer the nuts to a shallow baking dish or cookie sheet, and cool to room temperature before serving or storing. The nuts will keep for about 2 weeks in a resealable plastic bag in the refrigerator.

Serves 8.

Curried Almond Butter Dip

This creamy dip has a bit of a kick. It's a great dip or spread for fresh raw vegetables, adding a bit of protein to a light snack. This is best prepared in a smaller slow cooker, but you can double the recipe if you have a larger model.

- 2 cups almond butter
- 1 teaspoon mild curry powder, such as Madras
- 1/2 cup roasted almonds, finely chopped
- 1/4 cup white sesame seeds
- 1/2 cup unflavored almond milk

Combine all the ingredients in a large bowl and blend well with a mixing spoon. Pour the mixture into the slow cooker, cover, and cook on low heat for 4 hours. Pour into a shallow dish, cover, and refrigerate for at least 2 hours before serving. The dip will thicken as it cools.

Serves 8.

Herbed Meatballs

Meatballs are a classic party snack. Making them in the slow cooker is simple and easy to do in advance, freeing you up for other preparations. These meatballs freeze very well, too, if you'd like to save some for another meal.

- 2 pounds lean ground beef
- 1 large white onion, diced
- 1/2 cup chopped fresh parsley
- 1/4 cup chopped fresh basil
- 2 tablespoons chopped fresh oregano
- 1/2 cup almond meal
- 1 teaspoon sea salt
- 1/2 teaspoon freshly ground black pepper
- 2 large eggs, beaten

In a large mixing bowl, combine the beef, onion, parsley, basil, and oregano. Using clean hands, mix until well blended.

In a small bowl, combine the almond meal, salt, pepper, and eggs. Stir with a fork or whisk until blended. Pour over the meat and mix again with clean hands.

Form the mixture into 12 to 15 (2-inch) balls and place in the slow cooker in a single layer.

Cover and cook on low heat for 8 hours. To serve, place a toothpick in each meatball and arrange on a platter.

Serves 4.

Asian-Inspired Chicken Skewers

These delicious chicken skewers are reminiscent of your favorite Asian takeout, with flavors of nut butter, ginger, and scallions. They make a nice presentation for a casual dinner party and are a hit with kids.

- 3 pounds boneless, skinless chicken breasts (about 6 breasts)
- 1 teaspoon sea salt
- 1/2 cup sesame butter or tahini
- 1 teaspoon grated ginger
- 1/2 teaspoon red pepper sauce
- 12 bamboo skewers, soaked in water for 15 minutes
- 2 scallions, sliced

Using a sharp knife, butterfly the chicken breasts so that they are of even thickness, then slice each breast in half lengthwise. Season with the salt and set aside.

In a small bowl, thoroughly combine the sesame butter, ginger, and red pepper sauce. Pour the mixture into a gallon-sized resealable bag, add the chicken, and toss well to coat. Seal the bag and place on a flat surface in the refrigerator. Marinate for at least 3 hours or overnight, turning twice.

Thread 1 piece of chicken onto each bamboo skewer and place in the slow cooker. Pour the sesame butter mixture over the chicken, cover, and cook on low heat for 6 hours. To serve, place the skewers on a platter and garnish with the scallions.

Serves 6.

Slow Cooker Buffalo Drumettes with Paleo Ranch Dressing

One of the tenets of the Paleo diet is to choose lower-fat meats over the high-fat versions. However, it is acceptable to choose meats like chicken drumettes on a limited basis, and they make a wonderful, if rare, treat.

For the drumettes:

- 24 chicken drumettes, patted dry
- 1 cup red pepper sauce
- 2 tablespoons olive oil
- 1 teaspoon Worcestershire sauce
- 3 cloves garlic, crushed

For the Paleo ranch dressing:

- 1 cup coconut milk
- 1 cup Paleo-friendly mayonnaise
- 1/2 teaspoon garlic powder
- 1/2 teaspoon onion powder
- 1/2 teaspoon sea salt
- 1/2 cup fresh dill, chopped
- 1/4 cup fresh parsley, chopped

For serving:

- 2 fresh cucumbers, sliced
- 4 stalks celery, cut into 3-inch pieces

Make the drumettes:

Place the drumettes in a gallon-sized resealable plastic bag.

In a medium bowl, combine the red pepper sauce, olive oil, Worcestershire sauce, and garlic. Mix well with a fork and pour the mixture over the drumettes. Seal bag, shake well, and refrigerate for 1 hour.

Place the chicken with sauce into the slow cooker, cover, and cook on high heat for 4 hours.

Make the Paleo ranch dressing:

Combine the coconut milk, mayonnaise, garlic powder, onion powder, and salt, and mix well. Add the fresh herbs, stirring well. Chill for at least 1 hour.

To serve:

Place the drumettes on a platter, and serve the cucumber and celery on the side with small bowls of dressing.

Serves 4 to 6.

Slow-Cooked Baba Ghanoush

Baba ghanoush is a great change from the standard clam dip or other typical party spread. It's wonderful spread on Paleo-friendly crackers or used as a dip for fresh vegetables. This is a great recipe for when you have vegetarian guests, too.

- 2 medium eggplants, peeled
- 1 tablespoon paprika
- 1 tablespoon ground cumin
- 1 teaspoon freshly ground black pepper
- 4 cloves garlic, crushed
- 1/2 cup chopped fresh parsley, plus additional for garnish
- 2 tablespoons fresh lemon juice, divided
- 4 tablespoons tahini

Slice the eggplant into 1/2-inch slices and season each with the paprika, cumin, and pepper. Place 1 layer of eggplant into the slow cooker, and sprinkle with half of the garlic and half of the parsley.

Repeat with a second layer. Pour 1 tablespoon of the lemon juice over the eggplant, cover, and cook on low heat for 2 hours.

Transfer the eggplant to a large cutting board and cool for a few minutes. Place eggplant in a blender or food processor, add the tahini, and blend mixture until it is still chunky, but of a spreadable consistency.

Transfer the baba ghanoush to a shallow bowl, pour the remaining 1 tablespoon lemon juice over the top, and garnish with fresh parsley, if desired.

Serves 6.

All Day Pâté

Slow cooking the ingredients for this liver pâté allows the flavors to really develop. Classic pâtés are often refrigerated for days to allow flavors to mellow; slow cooking lets you skip that step with great results.

- 1 tablespoon olive oil
- 3 cloves garlic, crushed
- 1 medium onion, chopped
- 1/2 teaspoon sea salt
- 1/2 teaspoon freshly ground black pepper
- 1/2 teaspoon ground nutmeg
- 1/2 cup chopped fresh parsley
- 1 cup fresh mushrooms, roughly chopped
- 2 pounds beef liver, cut into 2-inch pieces

In a heavy skillet, heat the olive oil over medium heat. Add the garlic, onion, salt, pepper, nutmeg, parsley, and mushrooms, and sauté for 5 minutes, stirring frequently.

Add the liver to the pan, stirring well. Pour the mixture into the slow cooker, cover, and cook on low heat for 6 hours.

Transfer the mixture to a shallow dish and allow it to cool about 15 minutes, or until almost room temperature.

Place in a blender or food processor and blend until smooth. Scoop the pâté into a serving dish and refrigerate for 1 hour before serving. To serve, spread on Paleo-friendly crackers or toast points, or sliced hard-boiled eggs.

Serves 6.

Chili-Flavored Pumpkin Seeds

Pumpkin seeds are a deliciously crunchy-sweet snack. Traditionally roasted, these pumpkin seeds come out of the slow cooker with a delightfully warm kick that makes them great for eating out of your hand or for using as a topper for salads, soups, or baked sweet potatoes.

- 2 egg whites
- 1 teaspoon chili powder
- 1/2 teaspoon sea salt
- 1/4 teaspoon freshly ground black pepper
- 2 cups pumpkin seeds (raw but well dried)

In a large bowl, whisk the egg whites until foamy, then stir in the chili powder, salt, and pepper until well combined. Add the pumpkin seeds and toss well to coat.

Pour the pumpkin seeds into the slow cooker, cover, and cook on low heat for 4 hours. Transfer to a baking sheet to cool. Serve slightly warm or at room temperature. Store in the refrigerator in an airtight container for up to 1 week.

Serves 4 to 6.

Paleo Granola Bars

These granola bars cook up moist and flavorful in the slow cooker. Cut into bars for lunchtime snacks or a quick breakfast, or you can crumble them and top with almond milk for a great breakfast granola.

- 1/2 cup sesame butter
- 1/2 cup coconut oil, melted
- 1/4 cup raw honey
- 1 tablespoon pure vanilla extract
- 1 cup chopped raw almonds
- 1 cup chopped black walnuts
- 1 cup roasted pumpkin seeds
- 1/2 cup white sesame seeds
- 1 cup dried unsweetened cranberries
- 1 cup dried unsweetened apricots, chopped
- 1/2 cup unsweetened coconut flakes
- 2 cups almond flour
- 2 eggs, lightly beaten

In a medium saucepan, combine the sesame butter, coconut oil, honey, and vanilla. Warm over low heat, just until the oil and honey melt. Remove from heat and set aside.

In a large bowl, combine the almonds, walnuts, pumpkin seeds, sesame seeds, cranberries, apricots, and coconut. Toss well to blend. Add the almond flour and stir well, then add the eggs and stir well again.

Stir the honey mixture into the nut mixture and press into the bottom of the slow cooker. Cover and cook on low heat for 2 hours. Using a spatula, transfer the granola to a baking sheet and allow it to cool before cutting into bars. The bars will keep well in an airtight container in the refrigerator for up to 1 week.

Serves 12.

Stuffed Jalapeño Peppers

This snack is a great one for football Saturdays, backyard barbecues, and Tex-Mex nights with friends. If you like things a little fiery, leave some of the seeds in the jalapeños.

- 1 pound chicken sausage, casing removed
- 1 small onion, chopped
- 1/2 cup diced red bell pepper
- 8 fresh jalapeño peppers, halved and seeds removed

In a medium bowl, stir together the sausage, onion, and bell pepper until well blended. Divide the mixture between the pepper halves, spooning it in loosely.

Position the peppers in the bottom of the slow cooker. If you need to do two layers, rotate the second layer 90 degrees in a crosshatch pattern. Cover and cook on low heat for 4 hours. Arrange on a platter and serve slightly warm.

Serves 8.

SOUPS, STEWS, AND STOCKS

Steak and Sweet Roots Chili

Beans may be off-limits on the Paleo diet, but that doesn't mean you have to do without the great flavor of a hearty chili. This one uses carrots and sweet potatoes to stand in for the beans. It's so tasty that you'll never miss what's not there.

- 2 tablespoons olive oil
- 2 pounds top sirloin steak, cut into 1-inch pieces
- 4 sweet potatoes, peeled and cut into 1-inch pieces
- 4 carrots, peeled and cut into 1-inch pieces
- 2 (10-ounce) cans diced tomatoes with green chilies
- 1 large onion, chopped
- 1 red bell pepper, chopped
- 5 cloves garlic, crushed
- 2 (10-ounce) cans beef broth or 2 1/2 cups beef stock
- 1 tablespoon ground cumin
- 1 1/2 tablespoons chili powder
- Chopped green onions, for garnish

In a heavy skillet, heat the olive oil over medium-high heat. Add the steak (in batches, if necessary) and brown on all sides for 4 to 5 minutes.

Add all of the vegetables to the slow cooker, pour in the broth, and add the cumin and chili powder. Stir well to combine. Add the steak, cover, and cook on low heat for 8 hours.

To serve, ladle the chili into deep bowls and top with green onions.

Serves 8.

Italian Tomato Soup

When you want your tomato soup to have a little more gusto than the traditional cream variety, this recipe is sure to satisfy you. It's great as a starter or a light meal, and the combination of fresh and pantry ingredients makes it a great standby.

- 2 (15-ounce) cans whole tomatoes with juice
- 1 (15-ounce) can tomato sauce
- 3 1/2 cups chicken stock or broth
- 1 large white onion, chopped
- 2 cups fresh baby spinach leaves
- 3 cloves garlic, crushed
- 1 tablespoon chopped fresh basil
- 1 tablespoon chopped fresh oregano
- 1/2 teaspoon sea salt
- 1/4 teaspoon freshly ground black pepper

Add the tomatoes with juice, tomato sauce, and chicken broth to the slow cooker and stir well to combine. Add the onion, spinach, garlic, basil, and oregano, then season with salt and pepper, stirring well to incorporate.

Cover and cook on low heat for 4 hours. To serve, ladle the soup into deep bowls and serve with a green salad and Paleo-friendly crackers or bread.

Serves 10.

Creamy Mushroom Soup

On a brisk day or cool evening, nothing satisfies quite like a rich, creamy bowl of soup. This one is so much better for you than the canned variety, and the taste leaves no comparison. This soup doesn't freeze well, but you can make a big batch and store it in the fridge for up to a week.

- 2 tablespoons olive oil
- 8 ounces fresh white mushrooms, sliced
- 8 ounces fresh portobello mushrooms, sliced
- 1 small white onion, diced
- 1 clove garlic, crushed
- 1 teaspoon chopped fresh thyme
- 1 teaspoon chopped fresh rosemary
- 1 fresh or dried bay leaf
- 2 cups beef broth or stock
- 1/2 teaspoon sea salt
- 1/4 teaspoon freshly ground black pepper
- 1 cup coconut milk
- 1 teaspoon arrowroot powder
- Chopped fresh parsley, for garnish

In a large, heavy skillet, heat the olive oil over medium heat. Add the mushrooms, onion, and garlic, and sauté until the mushrooms are just browned and the onions are slightly translucent. Stir in the thyme, rosemary, and bay leaf, and cook for 1 more minute.

Transfer the mushroom mixture to the slow cooker, add the broth, and season with salt and pepper. Cover and cook on low heat for 4 hours. Remove the bay leaf.

Uncover the slow cooker and increase to high heat. In a small bowl, whisk together the coconut milk and arrowroot powder until the powder dissolves. When the soup begins to bubble, whisk in the milk mixture and cook for about 5 minutes, stirring frequently. When the soup has thickened, it is ready to serve.

To serve, ladle the soup into deep bowls and top with parsley.

Serves 8.

Hearty Beef and Cabbage Soup

This soup is especially filling and comforting. It's a great meal in a bowl for busy weeknights—just turn it on in the morning and come home to a wonderful-smelling pot of soup.

- 1 pound lean ground beef
- 2 cups chopped red cabbage
- 2 cups chopped green cabbage
- 1 large white onion, chopped
- 2 carrots, peeled and sliced
- 1 clove garlic, crushed
- 1 teaspoon paprika
- 1 teaspoon ground cumin
- 1/4 teaspoon celery seed
- 1 dry bay leaf
- 4 cups beef broth
- 1/2 teaspoon sea salt
- 1/4 teaspoon freshly ground black pepper

In a large, heavy skillet, cook the beef over medium-high heat just until browned, breaking it up with a spatula periodically until crumbly. Drain all but 1 teaspoon or so of the drippings and return the skillet to the heat.

Add the cabbages, onion, carrots, garlic, paprika, cumin, and celery seed, and cook for 2 minutes, stirring frequently.

Transfer the mixture to the slow cooker and add the bay leaf and broth. Season with salt and pepper. Cover and cook on low heat for 8 hours.

Ladle the soup into bowls and serve with crusty Paleo-friendly bread.

Serves 10.

Chicken and Mushroom Soup

This recipe uses cooked or leftover chicken breast to make it especially easy to prepare on busy mornings. You can sauté the aromatic vegetables the night before to make it even easier to get this soup cooking before you head out the door.

- 1 teaspoon olive oil
- 2 carrots, peeled and diced
- 1 medium white onion, diced
- 2 ribs celery, sliced
- 1 clove garlic, crushed
- 8 ounces white mushrooms, sliced
- 1 bay leaf
- 1 teaspoon dried thyme
- 1 teaspoon dried rosemary
- 4 cups chicken stock or broth
- 4 diced cooked chicken breasts (about 3 cups)
- 1/2 teaspoon sea salt
- 1/4 teaspoon freshly ground black pepper
- Chopped fresh parsley, for garnish

In a large, heavy skillet, heat the olive oil over medium-low heat. Add the carrots, onion, and celery. Cook for about 10 minutes, stirring occasionally, until the onions are slightly caramelized. Stir in the garlic, mushrooms, bay leaf, thyme, and rosemary, and cook for 2 minutes.

Transfer the mixture to the slow cooker. Add the stock, chicken, salt, and pepper. Cover and cook on low heat for 6 hours.

To serve, ladle the soup into deep bowls and garnish with fresh parsley.

Serves 6.

Pork and Sweet Potato Stew

This stew celebrates some of the classic flavors of fall and makes a deliciously comforting meal in cooler weather. Served with a green salad, it's a filling meal the whole family will enjoy.

- 1 pound lean pork stew meat
- 1/2 teaspoon sea salt
- 1/4 teaspoon freshly ground black pepper
- 1/2 teaspoon ground turmeric
- 1 teaspoon olive oil
- 1 medium white onion, chopped
- 4 sweet potatoes, peeled and cut into 1-inch pieces
- 3 parsnips, peeled and cut into 1-inch pieces
- 3 cups chicken broth or stock, divided
- 1 teaspoon chopped fresh rosemary
- 1 teaspoon chopped fresh tarragon
- 1/2 teaspoon arrowroot powder
- Fresh rosemary sprigs, for garnish

Trim the pork of visible fat and sinew. Cut meat into bite-size pieces and season with the salt, pepper, and turmeric.

In a large, heavy skillet, heat the olive oil over medium-high heat. Add the pork (in batches, if necessary) and brown on all sides for 3 to 4 minutes.

Place the onion, sweet potatoes, and parsnips in the slow cooker, pour in 2 1/2 cups of the broth, add the rosemary and tarragon, and stir well to combine. Add the pork, cover, and cook on low heat for 8 hours.

Uncover the slow cooker and increase to high heat. In a small bowl, whisk together the remaining 1/2 cup broth and arrowroot powder until the powder dissolves. Whisk the mixture into the stew and stir frequently for about 10 minutes, or until thickened nicely.

To serve, ladle the stew into shallow bowls and garnish with a rosemary sprig.

Serves 10.

Farmhouse Chicken and Vegetable Soup

This chicken and vegetable soup celebrates the simple yet delicious flavors of the garden. It's a classic soup that's filled with old-fashioned comfort-food goodness. It freezes very well, so make this big batch recipe and store some for another day.

- 8 boneless, skinless chicken thighs
- 1/2 teaspoon sea salt
- 1/4 teaspoon freshly ground black pepper
- 1 teaspoon olive oil
- 4 carrots, peeled and sliced
- 1 large white onion, chopped
- 2 stalks celery, sliced
- 1 tablespoon chopped fresh rosemary
- 1/2 teaspoon dried sage
- 1/4 cup chopped fresh flat-leaf parsley
- 1 bay leaf
- 6 cups chicken broth or stock

Trim the chicken of any visible fat. Cut meat into 1/2-inch strips, and season with the salt and pepper.

In a large, heavy skillet, heat the olive oil over medium-high heat. Add the chicken (in batches, if necessary) and brown on all sides for about 2 minutes. Transfer to the slow cooker with a slotted spoon, leaving about 1 teaspoon of the drippings in the skillet. Reduce the heat to medium; add the carrots, onion, and celery; and cook for 3 minutes, stirring frequently. Transfer to the slow cooker.

Stir in the rosemary, sage, parsley, bay leaf, and broth. Cover and cook on low heat for 8 hours.

Ladle the soup into deep bowls and serve with a green salad and Paleo-friendly rolls.

Serves 8.

Mediterranean Beef Stew

This hearty beef stew has a rich tomato sauce seasoned with basil and oregano, giving it a taste of the Mediterranean. Serve it with an arugula salad or some roasted endive for a meal that tastes like you're on vacation.

- 1 1/2 pounds lean beef stew meat
- 1/2 teaspoon sea salt
- 1/2 teaspoon freshly ground black pepper
- 1 teaspoon olive oil
- 8 ounces portobello mushrooms, sliced
- 1 cup fresh baby spinach leaves
- 1 cup frozen pearl onions, thawed
- 2 cups beef broth or stock, divided
- 1 (28-ounce) can crushed tomatoes with juice
- 1 (6-ounce) can tomato paste
- 2 cloves garlic, crushed
- 1 tablespoon chopped fresh basil
- 1 tablespoon chopped fresh oregano
- 1 teaspoon arrowroot powder

Trim the beef of any visible fat and cut into bite-size pieces. Season with the salt and pepper.

In a large, heavy skillet, heat the olive oil over medium-high heat. Add the beef (in batches, if necessary) and brown on all sides for 5 to 6 minutes.

Place the mushrooms, spinach, and pearl onions into the slow cooker. Add the meat.

In a medium bowl, stir together 1 3/4 cups broth, tomatoes with juice, tomato paste, garlic, basil, and oregano. Pour over the meat and vegetables, cover, and cook on low heat for 7 to 8 hours, or until the beef is tender.

Uncover the slow cooker and increase to high heat. In a small bowl, whisk together the remaining 1/4 cup broth and arrowroot powder until the powder dissolves. Stir into the stew and cook for about 5 minutes, stirring frequently, until slightly thickened.

To serve, ladle the stew into shallow bowls and top with Paleo-friendly croutons.

Serves 6.

Slow Cooker Beef Stew

There are few things that say "comfort food" better than a hearty beef stew. Slow cooking means the meat is always succulent and tender, plus your home is filled with wonderful aromas.

- 1 1/2 pounds lean beef stew meat
- 1/2 teaspoon sea salt
- 1/2 teaspoon freshly ground black pepper
- 1 teaspoon olive oil
- 4 carrots, peeled and cut into 1-inch pieces
- 1 stalk celery, sliced
- 1 large onion, roughly chopped
- 1 bunch fresh kale, trimmed and roughly chopped
- 1 bay leaf
- 1/4 cup chopped fresh parsley
- 3 cups beef broth or stock, divided
- 1 teaspoon arrowroot powder

Trim the beef of any visible fat. Cut the meat into bite-size pieces, and season with the salt and pepper.

In a large, heavy skillet, heat the olive oil over medium-high heat. Add the beef (in batches, if necessary) and brown on all sides for 4 to 5 minutes.

Add the carrots, celery, onion, kale, bay leaf, and parsley to the slow cooker, then add the beef. Pour 2 3/4 cups of the broth over the meat and vegetables. Cover and cook on low heat for 8 hours.

Uncover the slow cooker and increase to high heat. In a small bowl, whisk together the remaining 1/4 cup broth and arrowroot powder until the powder dissolves. Stir into the stew and cook for about 5 minutes, stirring frequently, just until thickened.

Ladle the stew into shallow bowls and serve with a fresh salad and Paleo-friendly bread.

Serves 6.

Garden Vegetable Soup

If you have your own vegetable garden, you have a thousand different recipes for vegetable soup at your fingertips; just pick whatever happens to be ripe and let the slow cooker blend the flavors beautifully. If you don't grow your own veggies, farmers' markets are great places to pick up the season's best ingredients.

- 1 teaspoon olive oil
- 1 stalk celery, sliced very thinly
- 1 carrot, peeled and sliced very thinly
- 1 medium white onion, diced
- 1/2 teaspoon sea salt
- 1/4 teaspoon freshly ground black pepper
- 1 teaspoon fresh oregano, chopped
- 1 teaspoon fresh basil, chopped
- 1/4 cup fresh parsley, chopped
- 1 medium zucchini, cut into 1-inch chunks
- 3 yellow squash, cut into 1-inch chunks
- 2 cups fresh baby spinach leaves
- 4 plum tomatoes, diced
- 4 cups vegetable or chicken broth
- 1 (6-ounce) can tomato paste

In a large, heavy skillet, heat the olive oil over medium heat. Add the celery, carrots, onion, salt, and pepper, and sauté for 5 minutes. Transfer the mixture to the slow cooker. Stir in the oregano, basil, and parsley. Add the zucchini, squash, spinach, and tomatoes, and stir well.

In a medium bowl, combine the broth and tomato paste, and stir with a fork just until blended. Pour over the vegetables, cover, and cook on high heat for 4 hours.

Ladle the soup into deep bowls and serve with crusty Paleo-friendly bread or crackers.

Serves 6.

Creamy Curried-Chicken Soup

This slightly exotic soup incorporates wonderful flavors from the East and is a great dish to make ahead for dinner guests. It tastes like you cooked all day, and you don't have to tell your guests you weren't home at the time.

- 2 pounds boneless, skinless chicken thighs
- 1 teaspoon olive oil
- 1 medium onion, diced
- 2 carrots, peeled and thinly sliced
- 1 tablespoon plus 1 1/2 teaspoons mild curry powder (such as Madras), divided
- 1 clove garlic, crushed
- 1/2 cup chopped fresh cilantro
- 1 small head cauliflower, cut into bite-size pieces
- 3 cups chicken broth or stock
- 1 cup coconut milk, divided
- 1/4 cup unsweetened coconut flakes
- 1 teaspoon arrowroot powder

Trim the chicken of visible fat and cut into 1-inch pieces.

In a large, heavy skillet, heat the olive oil over medium heat. Sauté the onion and carrots for 5 minutes. Stir in 1 tablespoon plus 1/2 teaspoon of the curry powder, garlic, cilantro, and cauliflower, and sauté for 2 minutes, stirring frequently.

Transfer the mixture to the slow cooker and add the chicken, broth, and 3/4 cup of the coconut milk. Stir well to combine, cover, and cook on low heat for 4 hours.

In a small, heavy skillet, combine the remaining 1 teaspoon curry powder with the coconut flakes and toast over medium-high heat for about 3 minutes, just until golden. Set aside.

Uncover the slow cooker and increase to high heat. In a small bowl, whisk together the remaining 1/4 cup coconut milk and arrowroot powder until the powder dissolves. Stir into the soup and cook for about 5 minutes, stirring frequently, until slightly thickened.

To serve, ladle the soup into shallow bowls and top each portion with some of the curried coconut.

Serves 8.

Pork and Butternut Squash Soup

Preparing the butternut squash two ways lends an extra depth of flavor to this creamy soup. If you'll be away from home while this cooks, prepare the roasted squash the night before and just store it in the fridge. Simply reheat it in the microwave before proceeding.

- 2 large butternut squash, peeled and cut into 2-inch chunks, divided
- 1 teaspoon olive oil
- 1/2 teaspoon ground cinnamon
- 1 pound lean ground pork
- 1 small onion, diced
- 1 clove garlic, crushed
- 1/2 teaspoon ground turmeric
- 1/2 teaspoon ground coriander
- 1/2 teaspoon sea salt
- 1/4 teaspoon freshly ground black pepper
- 2 cups beef stock or broth
- 1 cup unflavored almond milk
- Freshly chopped parsley, for garnish

Preheat the oven to 375 degrees F.

Line a rimmed baking sheet with aluminum foil.

In a medium-sized bowl, toss half of the squash pieces with the olive oil and arrange in a single layer on the baking sheet. Sprinkle with the cinnamon and roast for 35 to 40 minutes, or until fork-tender. Cool to room temperature and store in the refrigerator until ready to use.

In a large heavy skillet, cook the pork over medium-high heat until browned. Drain the drippings. Return to heat and stir in the onion, garlic, turmeric, coriander, salt, and pepper. Cook for 2 more minutes, stirring frequently.

Place the uncooked squash pieces in the slow cooker, then stir in the meat mixture, stock, and almond milk. Cover and cook on low heat for 8 hours.

Place the warm roasted squash in a blender or food processor. Blend until thick and smooth. Stir into the slow cooker, cover, and continue to cook for 10 more minutes.

To serve, ladle the soup into deep bowls and garnish with fresh parsley.

Serves 4.

Zucchini Soup Provençal

This light soup is full of the flavors of a summer in Provence. It's a great way to make the most of summer produce, especially if you have a garden that's become overwhelmed with zucchini. This soup doesn't take as long as many slow cooker soups, so it's a good one to make while you're at home.

- 1 teaspoon olive oil
- 2 shallots, diced
- 1 clove garlic, crushed
- 2 carrots, peeled and thinly sliced
- 4 medium zucchini, peeled and diced
- 1/2 teaspoon sea salt
- 1/4 teaspoon freshly ground black pepper
- 4 plum tomatoes, diced
- 1/4 cup tomato paste
- 1 tablespoon herbes de Provence
- 3 cups chicken or vegetable broth
- 1 tablespoon light olive oil
- 1/2 cup Paleo-friendly croutons

In a large, heavy skillet, heat the olive oil over medium heat. Add the shallots, garlic, carrots, and zucchini, and sauté for 2 to 3 minutes, stirring frequently. Season with the salt and pepper and transfer to the slow cooker. Stir in the diced tomatoes with any juices.

In a medium bowl, whisk together the tomato paste, herbes de Provence, and broth just until blended. Pour over vegetables in the slow cooker, cover, and cook on low heat for 4 hours.

Transfer the soup to a heatproof dish and allow it to cool for 10 minutes. Place in a blender or food processor and blend the soup (in batches, if necessary) until smooth. The soup can be reheated in the microwave if it becomes too cool.

To serve, ladle the soup into deep bowls, drizzle each portion with 1/2 teaspoon of the light olive oil, and top with the croutons.

Serves 6.

Creamy Root Vegetable Soup

This smooth and creamy soup has just a touch of sweetness from a quick roasting of the vegetables. Feel free to roast them the night before while you're cooking something else. This soup is a huge hit with kids and others who don't typically like parsnips or turnips.

- 2 small turnips, peeled and diced
- 2 parsnips, peeled and diced
- 2 sweet potatoes, peeled and diced
- 2 carrots, peeled and diced
- 1 teaspoon olive oil
- 1/2 teaspoon sea salt
- 1/4 teaspoon freshly ground black pepper
- 1 medium sweet onion, such as Walla Walla or Vidalia, diced
- 1/2 teaspoon dried rosemary
- 1/4 teaspoon dried sage
- 1/4 teaspoon ground nutmeg
- 1 bay leaf
- 2 cups chicken broth or stock
- 1 cup unflavored almond milk
- Sprigs of fresh rosemary, for garnish

Preheat the oven to 375 degrees F.

Line a rimmed baking sheet with aluminum foil.

In a large bowl, combine the turnips, parsnips, sweet potatoes, and carrots, tossing to mix. Add the olive oil and toss to coat evenly. Spread the vegetables in a single layer on the baking sheet and season with the salt and pepper. Roast for 10 to 12 minutes, or just until they begin to color.

Transfer the vegetable mixture to the slow cooker and add the onion, rosemary, sage, nutmeg, bay leaf, and broth. Cover and cook on low heat for 4 hours.

Transfer the soup to a heatproof dish and allow it to cool for 10 minutes. Place in a blender or food processor and blend the soup (in batches, if necessary) until smooth. Return the blended soup to the slow cooker.

Meanwhile, heat the almond milk in the microwave until just warm. Stir into the soup, cover, and cook for 5 to 7 minutes, or until heated through.

To serve, ladle the soup into deep bowls and garnish with a rosemary sprig.

Serves 4.

Portuguese-Style Venison Stew

There is a wonderful Portuguese recipe for lamb shanks in a red wine sauce that is heavenly, but lamb is usually excluded from Paleo kitchens. This recipe uses much leaner venison, which becomes quite tender in the slow cooker.

- 2 pounds lean venison roast, such as loin
- 1/2 teaspoon freshly ground black pepper
- 1 teaspoon sea salt, divided
- 1 tablespoon olive oil
- 6 cloves garlic, chopped
- 1 large yellow onion, roughly chopped
- 4 carrots, peeled and cut into 1-inch pieces
- 1 (26-ounce) can whole tomatoes with juice
- 1 (6-ounce) can tomato paste
- 2 cups beef broth or stock
- 1 teaspoon dried rosemary
- 1 teaspoon dried thyme

Trim the venison of any visible fat and cut into bite-size pieces. Season with pepper and 1/2 teaspoon of the salt.

In a large, heavy skillet, heat the olive oil over medium-high heat. Add the venison (in batches, if necessary) and brown on all sides for 3 to 4 minutes. Remove from the skillet and set aside. Add the garlic, onion, and carrots to the skillet and cook, stirring frequently, for 3 to 4 minutes, adding additional olive oil if needed.

Transfer the vegetables to the slow cooker and stir in the venison. Pour in the tomatoes with juice, tomato paste, and broth, and stir well to blend. Add the salt, rosemary and thyme, and stir again. Cover and cook on low heat for 10 hours.

To serve, ladle the stew onto a rimmed plate and pour some of the braising liquid over the top. This is wonderful served with a fresh salad or sautéed leafy greens.

Serves 4.

Homemade Beef Stock

Although soup bones can be found in the freezer section of most supermarkets, it's best to use fresh ones. Buy soup bones and marrow bones, or ask your butcher for the less expensive neck, knuckle, and foot bones. You may get a great deal. (Sometimes they even give them away for free!)

- 2 pounds beef marrow, soup, or other meaty bones
- 1 small yellow onion, peeled and halved
- 1 stalk celery, leaves removed
- 2 carrots, peeled and halved
- 6 cups water

Preheat the oven to 400 degrees F.

Place the bones in 1 (or more) glass or stoneware baking dish. If using marrow bones, place them marrow side up. Roast the bones for 30 minutes. Using tongs, transfer them carefully to the slow cooker. Add the onion, celery, and carrots, and pour the water over the top.

Cover and cook on low heat for 10 to 12 hours, or until the stock reaches the desired depth of flavor. Strain into a large bowl or dish, discarding the solids.

Allow the stock to cool to room temperature before storing in the refrigerator in an airtight container. Let the stock chill overnight, then skim the fat from the top and divide into individual storage containers, if desired. The stock can be stored in the refrigerator for up to 1 week, or in the freezer for 6 months.

Makes about 1 quart.

Homemade Beef Broth

Beef broth doesn't need to be cooked quite as long as beef stock in order to be delicious, and there are no hard-and-fast rules on seasonings, but you may want to be cautious when using strongly flavored herbs and spices.

- 2 pounds beef marrow bones or soup bones, or other meaty bones
- 1/2 teaspoon sea salt
- 1/4 teaspoon freshly ground black pepper
- 1/4 cup chopped onion
- 1/4 cup carrot, peeled and diced
- 1 stalk celery, halved
- 1 bay leaf
- 1 tablespoon chopped fresh parsley
- 6 cups water

Preheat the oven to 400 degrees F.

Place the bones in 1 (or more) glass or stoneware baking dish. If using marrow bones, place them marrow side up. Season the bones with salt and pepper and roast for 30 minutes. Using tongs, transfer them carefully to the slow cooker. Add the onion, carrot, celery, bay leaf, and parsley, then pour the water over the top.

Cover and cook on low heat for 6 hours. Strain into a large bowl or dish, discarding the solids.

Allow the broth to cool to room temperature before storing in the refrigerator in an airtight container. Let the broth chill overnight, then skim the fat from the top and divide into individual storage containers, if desired. The broth can be stored in the refrigerator for up to 1 week, or in the freezer for 6 months.

Makes about 1 quart.

Homemade Chicken Stock

This recipe calls for making the most of a leftover chicken carcass once you've carved the meat from it. It's a great way to stretch your food budget and delivers a remarkably tasty batch of stock. If you'd like to make a broth, add some salt, pepper, bay leaf, rosemary, and thyme before slow cooking.

- 1 carcass from a whole cooked chicken, with some meat remaining
- 1 small yellow onion, peeled and halved
- 1 stalk celery, leaves removed
- 2 carrots, peeled and halved
- 6 cups water

Place the chicken and vegetables in the slow cooker and pour in the water. Cover and cook on low heat for 6 hours. Remove the carcass and strain the stock into a large bowl or dish, discarding the solids.

Allow the stock to cool to room temperature before storing in the refrigerator in an airtight container. Let the stock chill overnight, then skim the fat from the top and divide into individual storage containers, if desired. The stock can be stored in the refrigerator for up to 1 week, or in the freezer for 6 months.

Makes about 1 quart.

Homemade Vegetable Stock

*Although the Paleo diet is certainly meat friendly, a vegetable stock is
sometimes better for recipes that call for a light flavor. It's also nice to have
on hand for vegetarian family members or guests. Almost any vegetable scrap
can go into a stock, so toss them into a resealable bag in the freezer as you
cook other meals until you are ready to make your stock. You should avoid
cabbage, broccoli, Brussels sprouts, and cauliflower, though, as they impart
too assertive a flavor.*

- At least 4 cups assorted raw vegetable scraps, such as carrot tops and tips, celery and onion trimmings, squash caps and ends, and so on
- 1 tablespoon olive oil
- 8 cups water (or 2 cups water for every 1 cup vegetables)

Preheat the oven to 375 degrees F.

Line a rimmed baking sheet with aluminum foil.

In a large bowl, toss the vegetable cuttings with the olive oil. Arrange
the vegetables on the baking sheet and roast for 15 minutes.

Transfer to the slow cooker, add water, and cook on low heat for 8 hours.
Strain the stock into a large bowl or dish, discarding the solids.

Allow the stock to cool to room temperature before storing in the
refrigerator in an airtight container. Let the stock chill overnight, then
divide into individual storage containers, if desired. The stock can be
stored in the refrigerator for up to 1 week, or in the freezer for 1 year.

Makes about 2 quarts.

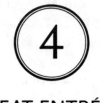

MEAT ENTRÉES

Eye of Round Roast with Mustard Sauce

Eye of round roast is a lean cut of beef, so it tends to shrink mercilessly when roasted. In the slow cooker, however, it comes out juicy and tender without a lot of shrinking. Cutting roasts in half helps them cook more evenly and fit into the slow cooker more easily.

- 1 teaspoon olive oil
- 1 (3- to 4-pound) eye of round roast, halved
- 1/2 teaspoon sea salt
- 1/2 teaspoon freshly ground black pepper
- 3 tablespoons brown mustard

- 1 teaspoon garlic powder
- 1/2 teaspoon paprika
- 1/4 teaspoon ground nutmeg
- 1 large yellow onion, sliced
- 1 cup beef stock or broth
- 1 bay leaf

In a large, heavy skillet, heat the olive oil over medium-high heat. Add the roast and brown on all sides, 3 to 4 minutes per side. Sprinkle the roast halves on all sides with the salt and pepper. Transfer the roast to the slow cooker.

Meanwhile combine the mustard, garlic powder, paprika, and nutmeg in a small bowl.

Arrange the onions around the roast. Using a spoon, spread the mustard sauce over the roast. Pour the stock around the roast and add the bay leaf. Cover and cook on high for 10 hours.

To serve, transfer the meat to a cutting board, slice, and arrange on a platter. Discard the bay leaf and ladle the sauce and onions over the sliced meat.

Serves 6.

Slow Cooker Paleo Pot Roast

Pot roasts have been a slow cooker staple since the slow cooker was invented. The slow, even cooking locks in the flavor of tougher cuts, while ensuring that the meat comes out fork-tender. Chuck roast is too fatty for all but the occasional Paleo meal, but a sirloin tip roast is just as tender when made in a slow cooker.

- 1 tablespoon olive oil
- 1 (3-pound) sirloin tip roast, halved
- 2 medium yellow onions, sliced
- 3 cloves garlic, chopped
- 1/4 cup sliced celery
- 2 1/4 cups beef broth, divided
- 2 tablespoons tomato paste
- 4 carrots, peeled and cut into 2-inch pieces
- 2 red bell peppers, cut into 2-inch pieces
- 1/2 teaspoon dried oregano
- 1/2 teaspoon freshly ground black pepper
- 1 bay leaf
- 1/2 teaspoon arrowroot powder
- 1/4 cup chopped fresh parsley, for garnish

In a large, heavy skillet, heat the olive oil over medium-high heat. Add the roast and brown on all sides, 4 to 5 minutes per side. Transfer the roast to the slow cooker, reserving the drippings in the skillet. Reduce to medium heat and add the onions, garlic, and celery to skillet. Sauté for 2 minutes, then transfer to the slow cooker.

In a medium bowl, combine 2 cups broth and the tomato paste with a fork, then pour over the roast. Arrange the carrots and peppers around the roast and sprinkle the oregano and pepper over everything. Add the bay leaf, cover, and cook on low heat for 6 hours.

Transfer the roast to a platter. Using a slotted spoon, arrange the vegetables around the roast. Cover with foil to keep warm.

Increase the slow cooker to high heat. In a small bowl, whisk together the remaining 1/4 cup of broth and arrowroot powder until the powder dissolves. Whisk into the slow cooker. Cook, uncovered, stirring occasionally, until a slightly thickened gravy forms, 10 to 15 minutes.

To serve, pour the gravy over the roast and garnish with fresh parsley.

Serves 6.

Autumn Harvest Sirloin Roast

Fall's root vegetables lend a slightly different flavor to the typical pot roast, and slow cooking enhances their natural sweetness. A touch of unsweetened apple cider makes the meat and its gravy especially delicious.

- 1 tablespoon olive oil
- 1 (3-pound) sirloin tip roast
- 4 carrots, peeled and cut into 1-inch pieces
- 4 parsnips, peeled and cut into 1-inch pieces
- 1 butternut squash, peeled and cut into 1-inch chunks
- 1/2 teaspoon freshly ground black pepper
- 1/2 teaspoon dried rosemary
- 1/2 teaspoon dried thyme
- 1 cup beef stock or broth
- 1/2 cup unsweetened apple cider, divided
- 1/2 teaspoon arrowroot powder

In a large, heavy skillet, heat the olive oil over medium-high heat. Add the roast and brown on all sides, 4 to 5 minutes per side.

Arrange the carrots, parsnips, and squash on the bottom of the slow cooker and season with the pepper and herbs. Position the roast on top of the vegetables. Add the broth and 1/4 cup of the apple cider, cover, and cook on low heat for 6 hours.

Transfer the roast to a cutting board, slice, and arrange on a platter. Using a slotted spoon, arrange the vegetables around the roast. Cover with foil to keep warm.

Increase the slow cooker to high heat. In a small bowl, whisk the remaining 1/4 cup of apple cider and arrowroot powder together, until the powder is fully dissolved. Whisk into the slow cooker. Cook uncovered, stirring occasionally, until slightly thickened, 10 to 15 minutes. Serve in a gravy boat alongside the roast and vegetables.

Serves 6.

Slow-Cooked Stuffed Cabbage Rolls

This recipe is similar to the traditional stuffed cabbage dishes of Germany and Hungary. The sauce is slightly sweet, with just a hint of nutmeg, and you'll never miss the rice that's traditionally included.

- 8 cups water
- 12 large green cabbage leaves, washed
- 1 large yellow onion, diced
- 2 cloves garlic, crushed
- 2 carrots, peeled and grated
- 1 teaspoon sea salt
- 1/4 teaspoon freshly ground black pepper
- 1 (14-ounce) can diced tomatoes
- 1 pound lean ground beef
- 1 pound lean ground pork
- 1 (14-ounce) can tomato sauce
- 2 (6-ounce) cans tomato paste
- 1/2 teaspoon ground nutmeg
- 1/2 teaspoon ground cardamom
- 1 teaspoon raw honey

In a large pot, bring water to a boil. Add the cabbage leaves and cook for 3 minutes. Drain and rinse with cool water until cool enough to handle. Pat dry and set aside.

In a large bowl, combine the onion, garlic, carrots, salt, pepper, and diced tomatoes, stirring until well blended. In a separate bowl, using clean hands or a sturdy spoon, combine the ground beef and ground pork. Add the ground meat to the vegetables, and mix thoroughly.

Divide the mixture evenly between the cabbage leaves, rolling them like an egg roll. Position the rolls in a single tight layer in the slow cooker, seam sides down.

In a medium bowl, combine the tomato sauce, tomato paste, nutmeg, cardamom, and honey. Pour the mixture over the cabbage rolls, cover, and cook on high heat for 1 hour. Reduce to low heat and cook for 4 more hours.

To serve, arrange the cabbage rolls on a platter and spoon the sauce over the top.

Serves 6.

Southwestern Beef Brisket

This brisket has a nice kick from chili powder, garlic, and cumin. It comes out fork-tender, and you can either slice and eat it as an entrée or shred it for lettuce wraps or omelets. This freezes well for up to three months, so have some now and freeze some to use on another busy night.

- 1 (3- to 3 1/2-pound) beef brisket, halved
- 1 teaspoon chili powder
- 1 teaspoon garlic powder
- 1 teaspoon ground cumin
- 1/2 teaspoon sea salt
- 1/2 teaspoon freshly ground black pepper
- 1/4 cup red wine (or 1/4 cup beef stock plus 1 tablespoon cider vinegar)

Trim the brisket of any visible fat and place on a baking sheet.

In a small bowl, combine the chili powder, garlic powder, cumin, salt, and pepper. Rub the mixture over all sides of the brisket. Cover with aluminum foil and let stand for 1 hour.

Place the brisket in the slow cooker and pour the wine over the top. Cover and cook on low heat for 12 hours or until fork-tender.

To serve, slice the brisket against the grain or shred and use in wraps, soup, or sandwiches.

Serves 8 to 10.

Cuban-Style Roast Pork

Cuban roast pork is justly famous for being one of the best dishes to come from Cuban kitchens. The distinctive mojo sauce and slow, even cooking is what makes it so phenomenal. You can buy bottled mojo sauce in some stores, but it's far better fresh.

- 1 teaspoon ground cumin
- 1 teaspoon dried oregano
- 1/2 teaspoon sea salt
- 1/2 teaspoon freshly ground black pepper
- 2 bay leaves, stems removed
- 8 cloves garlic, thinly sliced or minced
- 1/2 cup fresh orange juice (unsweetened store-bought juice is okay)
- 1/2 cup lime juice
- 1/2 cup olive oil
- 1 (4-pound) pork shoulder roast
- 2 large sweet onions, thinly sliced

In a blender, combine the cumin, oregano, salt, pepper, and bay leaves. Blend on high until smooth, making sure the bay leaves have been completely pulverized, with no large pieces remaining (they can pose a choking hazard). Add the garlic and citrus juices, and blend until smooth. With the blender on low, slowly pour the olive oil through the top and blend until fully incorporated.

Using a metal skewer or a clean meat thermometer, punch holes all over the top and sides of the roast and place in a shallow dish. Pour half of the mojo sauce over the pork, storing the rest in an airtight container in the refrigerator.

Turn the roast to distribute the sauce on all sides, then cover and refrigerate overnight, turning at least once.

Place the roast in the slow cooker and surround with the onions. Cover and cook on low heat for 6 hours. Turn the roast over, pour the remaining mojo sauce over the top, re-cover, and cook for 2 more hours, or until fork-tender.

Transfer the roast to a cutting board and allow it to rest. Increase to high heat and let the mojo sauce and onions cook, uncovered, for about 30 minutes, or until somewhat reduced.

Slice the pork, arrange in a shallow dish, and pour the sauce over the top. Serve on Paleo-friendly crusty bread, in lettuce wraps, or with fried plantains and a salad.

Serves 8 to 10.

Herb and Lemon Pork Loins

This delicious and earthy recipe uses two half loins, as they are typically easier to find and less expensive than whole loins. If you have a small family, cook one for tonight and save the other for making a quick soup or adding to a salad.

- 1 tablespoon olive oil
- 2 (1 1/2-pound) pork loins
- 1 teaspoon sea salt
- 1/2 teaspoon freshly ground black pepper
- 2 tablespoons dried rosemary
- 2 tablespoons dried tarragon
- 1 medium lemon, halved

In a large, heavy skillet, heat the olive oil over medium-high heat. Add the pork loins and brown on all sides, about 3 minutes per side. Remove loins from the pan and cool for a few minutes.

Season the loins with the salt and pepper on all sides. Combine the rosemary and tarragon in a small bowl and rub into the tops of both loins.

Place the pork loins in the slow cooker. Squeeze the juice of 1 lemon half over the pork loins. Slice the other half thinly and arrange on the top of the loins.

Cover and cook on high heat for 4 hours. Transfer to a platter with lemon slices intact and let the meat rest for 10 minutes before slicing. Serve with a salad or steamed fresh vegetables.

Serves 6.

Buffalo-Style Shredded Pork Wraps

Lunch can be a tough meal for Paleo folk, especially when the deli or fast-food restaurant is right around the corner. This recipe combines the saucy flavor of buffalo wings with the ease of a lettuce wrap to make lunch decisions much easier.

For the wraps:

- 1 cup red pepper sauce
- 1/2 cup olive oil
- 1 teaspoon raw honey
- 1 (1 1/2-pound) boneless pork butt or shoulder roast
- 12 large romaine lettuce leaves, washed and dried

For the Paleo ranch dressing:

- 1 cup coconut milk
- 1 cup Paleo-friendly mayonnaise
- 1/2 teaspoon garlic powder
- 1/2 teaspoon onion powder
- 1/2 teaspoon sea salt
- 1/2 cup fresh dill, chopped
- 1/4 cup fresh parsley, chopped

Make the wraps:

In a medium bowl, combine the red pepper sauce, olive oil, and honey, whisking with a fork until the honey is fully incorporated. Transfer half of the mixture to an airtight container and refrigerate; leave the other half in the bowl.

Place pork in the bowl, turning until all sides are coated. Cover and refrigerate for 2 hours or overnight, turning once.

Place the roast in the slow cooker, discarding the marinade. Cover and cook on low heat for 8 hours.

Transfer the roast to a cutting board or large dish and use two forks to shred the meat.

Make the Paleo ranch dressing:

Combine the coconut milk, mayonnaise, garlic powder, onion powder, and salt, and mix well. Add the fresh herbs, stirring well. Chill for at least 1 hour.

To serve:

To serve, heat the reserved buffalo-style sauce in the microwave for about 90 seconds and mix into the shredded pork to taste. Lay 2 romaine leaves of about the same size, 1 on top of the other. Place about 1/3 cup of the meat in the widest end of the leaves and add Paleo ranch dressing to taste. Roll up like a burrito and serve.

Serves 6.

Ginger-Garlic Pork Loin

The taste of this pork loin is similar to that of mu shu pork; in fact, wrapped in lettuce leaves, it makes a nice substitution for the sugar- and salt-laden restaurant version.

- 1/2 cup good, strong beef broth (if you must use stock, add 1 teaspoon sea salt)
- 1 teaspoon olive oil
- 1 tablespoon raw honey
- 6 cloves garlic, crushed
- 1 teaspoon freshly chopped ginger or jarred ginger slices
- 1 teaspoon apple cider vinegar
- 1 small sweet onion, diced
- 1/4 cup chopped fresh cilantro
- 1/4 teaspoon freshly ground black pepper
- 2 (1-pound) pork loins
- 6 large romaine lettuce leaves
- 8 scallions, sliced

In a blender or food processor, combine the broth, olive oil, honey, garlic, ginger, vinegar, onion, cilantro, and pepper. Blend on high until the mixture is opaque and the oil and honey are fully incorporated.

Pour the mixture into a shallow dish and add the pork loins, turning once to coat all sides. Cover and let stand for 1 hour, turning once.

Place the pork loins in the slow cooker and pour the marinade over the top. Cover and cook on high heat for 4 hours.

Remove the loins and allow them to rest for 10 minutes before slicing thinly. To serve, place 1/3 cup pork on the widest end of a lettuce leaf, spoon a bit of sauce over the meat, add a sprinkling of scallions, and roll up like a burrito.

Serves 6.

Split Roasted Lemon-Herb Chicken

This recipe takes some guidance from classic French recipes to turn an ordinary whole roasting chicken into something light, flavorful, and deliciously moist. If you live alone or are cooking for two, this can actually make a few small meals or snacks. Cooking it on a rack ensures that most of the chicken fat is left behind.

- 1 (3- to 3 1/2-pound) roasting chicken
- 8 sprigs fresh tarragon
- 4 sprigs fresh rosemary
- 4 sprigs fresh thyme
- 4 fresh sage leaves

- 2 (6-inch) lengths kitchen or butcher's twine
- 1 large lemon, sliced
- 1/2 teaspoon sea salt
- 1/2 teaspoon freshly ground black pepper

Place the chicken on a cutting board and cut in half lengthwise, using the breastbone as a guide. Loosen the skin along both breasts. Divide all of the herbs evenly into two bundles and tie tightly with the kitchen twine. Insert the herbs underneath the breast skin.

Insert half of the lemon slices underneath the skin and pull the skin so that it covers the lemon and herbs as completely as possible. Season each chicken half with the salt and pepper.

Place a small cake rack or several fist-sized bundles of foil in the bottom of the slow cooker and position the chicken halves on top. (It's okay if they overlap.) Cover and cook on high heat for 3 to 4 hours, or until a meat thermometer inserted into the thickest part of the thigh shows a temperature of at least 165 degrees F.

Transfer the chicken halves to a cutting board, allowing any fat to drip back into the slow cooker first. Remove the skin, herbs, and lemon slices; cut the chicken into serving portions; garnish with reserved lemon slices; and arrange on a platter.

Serves 4.

Tahini Chicken with Bok Choy

The food served at local Asian buffets and restaurants is often a no-no for anything other than a rare treat. This delicious recipe incorporates some of your favorite Asian restaurant flavors but skips all of the sugar, sodium, breading, and MSG.

- 3/4 cup tahini or sesame butter
- 2 tablespoons fresh lemon juice
- 1/2 teaspoon raw honey
- 1 teaspoon chopped fresh or jarred ginger
- 2 teaspoons chopped fresh cilantro
- 1/2 teaspoon sea salt
- 1/4 teaspoon freshly ground black pepper
- 1/2 teaspoon ground turmeric
- 3 cups roughly chopped bok choy
- 6 chicken breasts (about 2 pounds)
- 4 fresh scallions, sliced, for garnish

In a blender or food processor, combine the tahini, lemon juice, honey, ginger, cilantro, salt, pepper, and turmeric. Blend until smooth.

Place the bok choy in the slow cooker, making a bed for the chicken breasts. Spread a generous amount of the tahini mixture onto each chicken breast and arrange the breasts in a single layer over the bok choy. Cover and cook on low heat for 4 hours. To serve, garnish with fresh scallions.

Serves 6.

Chicken Breast Cacciatore

Chicken cacciatore is a classic Italian recipe that almost everyone enjoys. This is a great recipe to make for guests who are not on the Paleo diet. It's wonderful served with Paleo-friendly crusty bread and a romaine or arugula salad.

- 1 (28-ounce) can whole tomatoes
- 1 (6-ounce) can tomato paste
- 1/2 cup chicken stock
- 1 teaspoon chopped fresh oregano
- 1 teaspoon chopped fresh basil

- 6 cloves garlic, chopped
- 1 teaspoon sea salt
- 1/2 teaspoon freshly ground black pepper
- 6 chicken breasts (about 2 pounds)
- Chopped fresh parsley, for garnish

Using clean hands, remove the whole tomatoes from the can and squeeze them before placing in a medium bowl. Pour in the tomato juices. Stir in the tomato paste and stock, mixing well. Add the oregano, basil, garlic, salt, and pepper, and mix well.

Arrange the chicken breasts in a single layer in the slow cooker and pour the tomato mixture over the top. Cover and cook on low heat for 4 hours.

To serve, arrange the chicken breasts on a platter, pour sauce over the top, and garnish with fresh parsley. Serve the remaining sauce in a separate dish.

Serves 6.

Chicken and Mushrooms in Cream Sauce

This dish is pure comfort after a busy day. Coconut milk lends a delicious, slightly sweet taste. Fresh spinach and piles of mushrooms in a creamy sauce makes it a filling, satisfying meal that everyone will love, even the kids.

- 1 cup coconut milk, divided
- 1 cup chicken stock, divided
- 1/2 teaspoon sea salt
- 1/2 teaspoon freshly ground black pepper
- 1/2 cup chopped fresh parsley
- 2 tablespoons chopped fresh tarragon
- 1 teaspoon paprika
- 1 teaspoon olive oil
- 6 chicken breasts
- 1 small yellow onion, diced
- 2 cloves garlic, crushed
- 2 cups fresh baby spinach leaves
- 8 ounces white mushrooms, sliced
- 8 ounces portobello mushrooms, sliced
- 1 teaspoon arrowroot powder

In a blender, combine 3/4 cup of the coconut milk, 3/4 cup of the stock, salt, pepper, parsley, tarragon, and paprika. Blend just until smooth and set aside.

In a large, heavy skillet, heat the olive oil over medium-high heat. Add the chicken breasts and brown for 2 to 3 minutes on each side. Transfer to a plate.

Add the onion and garlic to the pan and cook, stirring often, for 2 to 3 minutes, or until the onions are just partly translucent. Increase the heat to high and carefully pour in the remaining 1/4 cup stock. Using a spatula or wooden spoon, quickly deglaze the pan by scraping up all of the brown bits. Add the spinach and mushrooms to the pan, and cook, stirring frequently, for 4 minutes.

Layer the chicken in the slow cooker, top with the mushroom mixture, and pour the blended mixture over the top. Cover and cook on low heat for 4 hours.

Transfer the chicken and vegetables to a platter. In a small bowl, whisk together the remaining 1/4 cup coconut milk with the arrowroot powder, until the powder is fully dissolved. Stir into the slow cooker and cook, uncovered, until the sauce is just thickened.

To serve, top the chicken and vegetables with sauce.

Serves 6.

Herb-Roasted Turkey Breast

Turkey is still wonderfully economical as far as meats go, making it a real lifesaver for the Paleo person on a tight budget. One whole turkey cut into several portions can provide you with many delicious meals. This recipe uses the lean breast for a flavorful entrée with delicious gravy.

- 1 (3-pound) turkey breast
- 1/2 teaspoon sea salt
- 1/2 teaspoon freshly ground black pepper
- 1/2 teaspoon dried sage
- 1/2 teaspoon dried thyme
- 1 teaspoon dried parsley
- 1 bay leaf
- 1 cup chicken stock, divided
- 1 teaspoon arrowroot powder

Season both sides of the turkey breast with the salt and pepper, then sprinkle the herbs all over the breast. Place the turkey breast in the slow cooker, add the bay leaf, and pour 3/4 cup of the stock over the top. Cover and cook on low heat for 6 hours.

Transfer the turkey to a cutting board and discard the skin.

Increase to high heat. In a small bowl, whisk together the remaining 1/4 cup stock with the arrowroot powder, until the powder is fully dissolved. Stir into the slow cooker and cook, uncovered, until slightly thickened, about 10 minutes.

To serve, slice the turkey breast and top with sauce.

Serves 6 to 8.

Walnut Turkey Breast with Root Vegetable Puree

This recipe is an elegant one to prepare for dinner guests. Have the butcher slice the turkey breast for you; most are happy to do so. If you can find the turnips with their greens intact, sauté the greens and serve on the side—they're delicious and one of the healthiest leafy greens.

- 6 pieces skinless turkey breast, sliced 1-inch thick
- 1 teaspoon walnut oil
- 1/2 teaspoon sea salt
- 1/4 teaspoon freshly ground black pepper
- 1 teaspoon dried thyme
- 1 teaspoon dried rosemary
- 1 teaspoon dried parsley
- 2 large turnips, peeled and diced
- 4 parsnips, peeled and sliced
- 4 carrots, peeled and sliced
- 1 cup chicken stock
- 1 teaspoon ground turmeric
- 1/2 cup chopped walnuts
- 6 sprigs fresh rosemary, for garnish

Pound the breasts, if necessary, to make sure that they are of even thickness.

In a large, heavy skillet, heat the walnut oil over medium-high heat. Season the turkey with the salt and pepper, and add to the skillet. Brown the turkey breasts for about 2 minutes on each side, taking care not to let the oil get too hot. Sprinkle the breasts with the thyme, rosemary, and parsley, and set aside.

Place the turnips, parsnips, and carrots in the slow cooker. Position the turkey breasts on top. Pour the stock over everything, cover, and cook on low heat for 4 hours.

Transfer the breasts to a platter and cover to keep warm.

Pour the contents of the slow cooker into a shallow dish and allow to cool for about 10 minutes. Add the turmeric and pour into a blender. Add the walnuts and blend just until smooth.

To serve, place a dollop of puree onto each plate, top with a turkey breast portion, and garnish with a rosemary sprig.

Serves 6.

Savory Herbed Turkey Drumsticks

Many Paleo followers try to abstain from poultry legs and wings the majority of the time. This recipe is an easy and very tasty one to prepare for those occasional treats.

- 4 turkey drumsticks, skin removed
- 1 tablespoon olive oil
- 1/2 teaspoon sea salt
- 1/2 teaspoon freshly ground black pepper
- 1 teaspoon dried parsley
- 1 teaspoon dried oregano

Rub the drumsticks with the olive oil until well coated, then sprinkle with the salt, pepper, parsley, and oregano.

Place the drumsticks in the slow cooker, cover, and cook on low heat for 8 hours.

To serve, place a drumstick on each plate and serve with a baked sweet potato, tossed salad, or roasted root vegetables.

Serves 4.

Turkey Legs with Kale

Kale is one of the most healthful green vegetables you can eat. Fortunately, it also tastes great. Slow cooking brings out its nutty flavor while ridding it of the slight bitterness. It's a perfect accompaniment to roasted turkey legs and needs no fancy seasoning.

- 2 bunches fresh kale, washed and ribs removed
- 1/2 teaspoon sea salt, divided
- 1/2 teaspoon freshly ground black pepper, divided
- 2 cups chicken stock
- 4 turkey drumsticks, skin removed
- 1 teaspoon walnut oil
- 1/2 teaspoon dried parsley
- 1/2 teaspoon paprika

Chop or tear the kale into large pieces, place in the slow cooker, and season with 1/4 teaspoon each of the salt and pepper. Pour the stock over the top.

Rub the drumsticks with the walnut oil, season with remaining 1/4 teaspoon each salt and pepper, and sprinkle with the parsley and paprika. Arrange on top of the kale, cover, and cook on low heat for 6 hours.

To serve, transfer the drumsticks to a platter. Using a slotted spoon, pile the kale around the drumsticks and pour the broth into a gravy boat for drinking or dipping bread.

Serves 4.

Venison Roast with Harvest Vegetables

Venison is very lean, but it's packed with rich flavor. It's become much easier to source venison, partly due to the popularity of the Paleo diet. If you've never tried it, this is a great recipe for your first experience.

- 1 (4-pound) venison roast, such as shoulder or loin, halved
- 1 teaspoon sea salt
- 1/2 teaspoon freshly ground black pepper
- 2 fresh sage leaves, chopped
- 1 tablespoon chopped fresh thyme
- 4 acorn squash, skin on, quartered
- 6 carrots, peeled and cut into 3-inch pieces
- 1 pound fresh Brussels sprouts, cores trimmed
- 1 teaspoon olive oil
- 1/2 teaspoon ground nutmeg

Trim any visible fat from the venison and season with the salt and pepper. Sprinkle with the sage and thyme and set aside.

In a large bowl, toss the squash, carrots, and Brussels sprouts with the olive oil and nutmeg. Place the vegetables in the slow cooker.

Arrange the roast on top of the vegetables, cover, and cook on high heat for 1 hour. Reduce to low heat and cook for 7 to 8 more hours, or until the venison is fork-tender.

Transfer the roast to a platter. Using a slotted spoon, arrange the vegetables around the venison and serve.

Serves 10.

Spicy Roast Venison

This is the perfect recipe for those who like their food just a little spicy. It's also a great way to cook a smaller venison roast.

- 1 (1-pound) venison roast, such as loin or shoulder
- 1 teaspoon chili sauce
- 1 teaspoon Worcestershire sauce
- 1 teaspoon raw honey
- 1 teaspoon ground cumin
- 1/2 teaspoon freshly ground black pepper

Trim any visible fat from the venison.

In a small bowl, combine the chili sauce, Worcestershire sauce, honey, cumin, and pepper, and rub all over the roast.

Place the roast in the slow cooker and cook on low heat for 4 hours, or until fork-tender.

Allow the roast to rest for 10 minutes. To serve, slice against the grain and arrange on a platter.

Serves 4.

Southern-Style Sausage and Collards

*Collard greens are wonderfully nutritious and have a savory flavor, but
they're not often prepared outside the South. Traditionally made with ham
hocks or bacon, this recipe uses fresh pork sausage to create a meal in a bowl
that's perfect for cool evenings.*

- 2 bunches collard greens (about 1 pound)
- 1 pound fresh uncured pork sausage, casing removed
- 1 large yellow onion, chopped
- 4 carrots, peeled and sliced
- 1/2 teaspoon sea salt
- 1/2 teaspoon cider vinegar
- 4 cups vegetable or chicken stock

Wash the collard greens very well to remove any grit, and cut out all of
the thicker ribs. Set aside in a colander to drain.

In a large, heavy stockpot, brown the sausage over medium heat, just
until lightly brown. Stir in the onion, carrots, and salt, and sauté for five
minutes. Stir in vinegar and stock, turn heat to high, and bring to a boil.

Add the collard greens to the pot, using a long spoon to push them
down after each addition. If necessary, wait a few minutes for them to
cook down a bit before adding more, as they'll be very bulky.

Once all the collards are incorporated, carefully pour all into the slow
cooker, cover, and cook on high for 4 hours.

To serve, spoon a generous portion of meat and vegetables into a bowl,
then ladle some of the broth over the top.

Makes 6 servings.

Spaghetti Squash with Chicken-Sausage Sauce

If you're missing your spaghetti with meatballs or sausage, you'll love this recipe. The sauce cooks all day, and you can roast the spaghetti squash during the last hour of cooking.

- 1 1/2 pounds uncured chicken sausage, sliced 1-inch thick
- 1 large yellow onion, diced
- 3 cloves garlic, crushed
- 1 (28-ounce) can tomato sauce
- 1 (6-ounce) can tomato paste
- 1 teaspoon Italian seasoning
- 1/2 teaspoon sea salt
- 1/4 teaspoon freshly ground black pepper
- 3 spaghetti squash, cut in half lengthwise, seeds removed
- 2 teaspoons olive oil, divided

In a large, heavy skillet, cook the chicken sausage over medium-high heat for about 5 minutes, stirring frequently to brown all of the pieces. Transfer to a paper towel and pat with another paper towel to remove excess grease.

Add the onion and garlic to skillet, and cook for 5 minutes, stirring frequently. Remove from the heat. Add the tomato sauce, tomato paste, Italian seasoning, salt, and pepper, and stir well.

Place the sausage in the slow cooker and pour the sauce over the top. Cover and cook on low heat for 6 hours.

During the last hour of cooking, preheat the oven to 375 degrees F.

Rub the spaghetti squash with 1 teaspoon of the olive oil and position cut side up on a baking sheet. Bake for 45 to 50 minutes, or until very tender.

Scoop the flesh out with a spoon into a large bowl. Drizzle with the remaining 1 teaspoon olive oil and toss well.

To serve, place a heaping portion of squash on a plate and ladle the chicken-sausage sauce over the top.

Serves 6.

VEGETARIAN ENTRÉES

Slow Cooker Ratatouille

This recipe is a riff on the classic French ratatouille, one of the most delicious ways to use the abundance of summer produce. The addition of walnuts makes it more filling and wonderfully different; you won't miss the traditional Parmesan topping.

- 1 tablespoon plus 1/2 teaspoon olive oil, divided
- 3 cloves garlic, crushed
- 2 large eggplants, cut into 1/2-inch slices
- 1 large red onion, cut into thin slices
- 2 yellow summer squash, cut into 1/2-inch slices
- 2 zucchini, cut into 1/2-inch slices
- 1/4 cup chopped fresh basil
- 1/4 cup chopped fresh oregano
- 1/4 cup chopped fresh parsley
- 1/2 teaspoon sea salt
- 1/2 teaspoon freshly ground black pepper
- 1/2 cup chopped walnuts

In a large, heavy skillet, heat 1 tablespoon of the olive oil over medium-high heat. Add the garlic and cook for 1 minute. Sauté the eggplant slices in batches for about 2 minutes per side. Transfer to paper towels to drain.

Pour the oil from the skillet into the slow cooker, and once slightly cooled, wipe around the crock to coat.

Place a layer of eggplant in the slow cooker and top with alternating slices of onion, squash, and zucchini. Season with half of the herbs, salt, and pepper. Repeat the layering with the remaining eggplant, vegetables, and seasonings. Cover and cook on high heat for 2 hours.

In a small skillet, heat the remaining 1/2 teaspoon olive oil and sauté the walnuts for 2 minutes, stirring frequently, just until they smell toasted. Remove from the heat.

To serve, plate each portion and top with the walnuts.

Serves 6.

No Parmesan Eggplant

This succulent eggplant casserole is a terrific Paleo-friendly substitute for traditional eggplant Parmesan, without all of the cheese. You won't even notice it's missing.

- 1 tablespoon olive oil
- 3 cloves garlic, crushed
- 1 large yellow onion, thinly sliced
- 4 medium eggplants, cut into 1-inch slices
- 1/2 teaspoon freshly ground black pepper
- 1 teaspoon sea salt, divided
- 1/2 teaspoon raw honey
- 1 (14-ounce) can crushed tomatoes
- 1 (14-ounce) can tomato sauce
- 1/2 teaspoon dried oregano
- 1/2 teaspoon dried basil
- 1/4 teaspoon celery seed

In a large, heavy skillet, heat the olive oil over medium heat. Sauté the garlic and onion for 3 to 4 minutes, or until the onions are translucent. Transfer to a small bowl and reserve.

Sauté the eggplant slices in batches for about 2 minutes per side. Season with pepper and 1/2 teaspoon of the salt. Layer the eggplant in the slow cooker. Once all of the eggplant is in the slow cooker, scatter the garlic and onions over the top.

In a medium bowl, combine the honey, tomatoes, tomato sauce, oregano, basil, celery seed, and remaining 1/2 teaspoon salt. Pour over the eggplant.

Cover and cook on low heat for 6 hours. To serve, place a portion of eggplant on a plate and spoon sauce over the top. Serve with a green salad and Paleo-friendly garlic bread.

Serves 6.

Vegetarian Collard Greens

Although traditional collard greens are typically seasoned using ham hocks or bacon, it is possible to make a delicious and satisfying pot of collards without using meat. For those meat-free days, or when you're cooking for a vegetarian friend or family member, this is the perfect dish.

- 2 bunches collard greens, ribs removed
- 3 cups vegetable stock
- 1 teaspoon sea salt
- 1/2 teaspoon freshly ground black pepper
- 1 teaspoon apple cider vinegar
- 4 carrots, peeled and cut into 1-inch pieces
- 2 sweet potatoes, cut into 1-inch pieces

Roughly chop or tear the collards into large pieces and rinse very well; drain.

Pour the stock into the slow cooker and add the salt, pepper, and vinegar. Add the carrots and sweet potatoes and top with the collard greens. You may have to pack them down, but they will eventually cook down enough to be submerged in the stock. Cover and cook on high heat for 4 hours or on low for 6 hours.

To serve, ladle the collard greens into deep bowls, adding some broth on top.

Serves 6.

Mixed Greens with Turnips

Mustard and turnip greens have distinctly different (but equally delicious) flavors. Using both the tops and the roots of the turnips is economical and makes the most of a wonderful vegetable.

- 4 turnips, greens attached
- 1 bunch mustard greens
- 1 bunch kale
- 2 teaspoons olive oil, divided
- 2 cloves garlic, crushed
- 1 medium sweet onion, diced
- 1/2 teaspoon sea salt
- 1/4 teaspoon freshly ground black pepper
- 1/2 teaspoon apple cider vinegar
- 2 cups vegetable broth

Wash the turnips and cut the greens from the tops. Chop the greens roughly and dice the roots, placing them in separate dishes.

Wash the mustard greens and kale and remove the ribs before chopping roughly. Place all of the greens (including turnip) in the slow cooker.

In a large, heavy skillet, heat 1 teaspoon of the olive oil over medium heat. Sauté the garlic and onion for 2 minutes. Add the turnips and sauté for 2 more minutes, stirring frequently.

Add the turnip mixture to the slow cooker, season with the salt and pepper, and add the vinegar. Pour the broth over the top, cover, and cook on high heat for 4 hours or low for 6 hours.

To serve, ladle into bowls with the broth, and top each portion with a drizzle of the remaining 1 teaspoon olive oil.

Serves 6.

Vegetarian Beanless Chili

It can be hard to find a good vegetarian chili recipe that isn't loaded with beans but is still hearty enough for a meal. This one fits that bill beautifully. Top with some crumbled Paleo-friendly crackers and you have a great dish that's perfect for lunch or dinner.

- 2 medium zucchini, cut into 1-inch pieces
- 2 summer squash, cut into 1-inch pieces
- 1 large eggplant, cut into 1/2-inch pieces
- 2 parsnips, peeled and cut into 1/2-inch pieces
- 2 carrots, peeled and cut into 1/2-inch pieces
- 2 medium yellow onions, chopped
- 2 stalks celery, thinly sliced
- 4 cups vegetable broth, divided
- 1 teaspoon ground cumin
- 1 teaspoon chili powder
- 1/4 cup chopped fresh cilantro
- 1/2 teaspoon sea salt
- 1/2 teaspoon freshly ground black pepper
- 1 teaspoon arrowroot powder

Put all of the vegetables into the slow cooker and pour 3 3/4 cups of the broth over the top. Add the cumin, chili powder, cilantro, salt, and pepper. Cover and cook on high heat for 4 hours.

In a small bowl, whisk together the remaining 1/4 cup broth and arrowroot powder until the powder dissolves completely. Stir into the chili and cook, uncovered, stirring occasionally, until thickened, 15 to 20 minutes.

Serves 6.

Fall Vegetable and Apple Stew

This recipe can make a nice vegetarian main dish or a tasty side for a pork or chicken dinner. Choose tart, firm apples like Fuji or Winesap for the best flavor and consistency.

- 2 sweet potatoes, peeled and cut into 1-inch pieces
- 4 carrots, peeled and cut into 1-inch pieces
- 4 parsnips, peeled and cut into 1-inch pieces
- 1 small yellow onion, diced
- 4 tart apples, cored, peeled, and thickly sliced
- 1/2 teaspoon sea salt
- 1/2 teaspoon freshly ground black pepper
- 1/2 teaspoon curry powder
- 1/2 teaspoon ground cinnamon
- 3 cups vegetable broth, plus 2 tablespoons (optional)
- 1/2 teaspoon arrowroot powder (optional)
- 1/2 cup pecan halves
- 1/2 cup chopped fresh parsley, for garnish

Put all of the vegetables and apples into the slow cooker and season with the salt, pepper, curry powder, and cinnamon. Pour the broth over the top, cover, and cook on low heat for 4 hours.

If the stew broth isn't thick enough for your liking, in a small bowl, whisk together 1/2 teaspoon arrowroot powder and 2 tablespoons vegetable broth until the powder dissolves. Stir into the stew and cook, uncovered, for about 15 minutes.

To serve, ladle the stew into deep bowls, sprinkle with the pecans, and garnish with fresh parsley.

Serves 6.

Portobello Mushroom Steaks

Portobello mushrooms have long been considered the vegetarian's rib-eye steak. They're succulent and meaty, with a consistency very much like beef. This recipe is a great vegetarian entrée, or a terrific side dish for an actual steak.

- 6 large portobello mushroom caps
- 1 tablespoon plus 1 teaspoon olive oil
- 1/2 teaspoon sea salt
- 1/2 teaspoon freshly ground black pepper

- 1 medium yellow onion, thinly sliced
- 1 red bell pepper, sliced
- 2 cloves garlic, crushed
- 1 tablespoon chopped fresh parsley
- 3 scallions, sliced

Slice the mushrooms into 2 or 3 thick slices per cap, about 3/4-inch thick. Toss in a large bowl with 1 tablespoon of the olive oil and season with the salt and pepper.

In a large, heavy skillet, heat the remaining 1 teaspoon olive oil over medium heat. Add the onions, bell pepper, and garlic, and sauté for 2 minutes.

Place the mushrooms in the slow cooker in a single layer (overlapping a bit is fine) and top with the onion mixture and parsley. Cover and cook on low heat for 2 hours.

To serve, place 4 to 5 mushroom slices on a plate, top with the onion mixture, and garnish with scallions.

Serves 4.

Thai-Style Vegetable Noodles

When you're craving pad Thai or a nice bowl of udon noodles, try this recipe on for size. It's packed with flavor and completely Paleo friendly and vegetarian. The veggie mixture tastes even better the second day. Store it separately from the spaghetti squash and reheat for a great work lunch.

- 1 1/2 cup dried shiitake mushrooms
- 1/2 cup vegetable broth
- 1 cup tahini
- 2 tablespoons crushed garlic
- 1 teaspoon raw honey
- 2 teaspoons red pepper sauce (or Louisiana hot sauce)
- 1/2 cup bamboo shoots

- 2 medium red onions, thinly sliced
- 2 yellow or orange bell peppers, thinly sliced
- 1 head bok choy, roughly chopped
- 2 spaghetti squash, halved lengthwise
- 4 scallions, sliced, for garnish

In a medium bowl, soak the shiitake mushrooms in the broth for 30 minutes to 1 hour, or until pliable. Carefully remove from the broth, squeezing excess liquid back into the bowl. Set the mushrooms aside.

Add the tahini, garlic, honey, and red pepper sauce to the broth, and stir well. Add the bamboo shoots, onion, bell pepper, bok choy, and mushrooms to the tahini mixture. Scoop into 1 side of the slow cooker. On the other side, place the squash, cut side up. (It's fine if they overlap a bit.)

Cover and cook on low heat for 3 hours, or until the squash is fork-tender. Remove the squash and use a spoon to scoop out the flesh into a large bowl. Pour the contents of the slow cooker over the top.

To serve, place a heaping portion in a shallow bowl and top with scallions.

Serves 4.

Vegetable Curry

Curry doesn't always have to include meat. This one is thick, rich, hearty, and full of flavor. It's even better the next day, so cook ahead if you can or save some of it for tomorrow's lunch.

- 2 cups vegetable stock
- 1 cup coconut milk, divided
- 1/2 teaspoon sea salt
- 1/2 teaspoon freshly ground black pepper
- 1 to 2 teaspoons of mild curry powder (to taste)
- 1/2 teaspoon ground nutmeg
- 2 medium yellow onions, chopped
- 1 large zucchini, cut into chunks
- 3 carrots, peeled and cut into thick slices
- 1 butternut squash, cut into 1-inch chunks
- 1 teaspoon arrowroot powder
- 1/2 cup chopped fresh chives

Combine the stock, 3/4 cup of coconut milk, salt, pepper, curry powder, and nutmeg in the slow cooker and stir well. Add all of the vegetables, cover, and cook on low heat for 6 hours.

Increase to high heat. In a small bowl, whisk together the remaining 1/4 cup coconut milk and arrowroot powder until the powder dissolves. Stir into the curry and cook, uncovered, until thickened, about 15 minutes.

To serve, ladle the curry into deep bowls and top with chives.

Serves 6.

Stuffed Acorn Squash

The pecans and mushrooms in this recipe play beautifully on the nutty flavor of the acorn squash. Served with a spinach and tomato salad, this makes a light but satisfying meal.

- 2 acorn squash, halved lengthwise and seeds removed
- 1 teaspoon walnut oil
- 1 pound portobello mushrooms, chopped
- 1 medium yellow onion, diced
- 2 cloves garlic, crushed
- 2 cups fresh baby spinach leaves
- 1/2 cup chopped pecans
- 1 teaspoon paprika
- 1/2 teaspoon sea salt
- 1/4 teaspoon freshly ground black pepper
- 1/2 teaspoon ground nutmeg

Use a fork to make several shallow holes in each squash half, and place each half cut side up in the slow cooker.

In a medium-sized, heavy skillet, heat the walnut oil over medium heat. Add the mushrooms, onion, garlic, spinach, and pecans, and stir well. Sprinkle the paprika, salt, pepper, and nutmeg over the top, and sauté for about 2 minutes, stirring frequently.

Divide the mixture between the squash halves. Cover and cook on low heat for 6 hours.

Serves 4.

BREADS AND DESSERTS

Slow Cooker Banana Bread

If you're lucky enough to be home when this bread is baking, the smell will drive you wild! Full of ripe bananas and scented with vanilla, you'd never know this banana bread is actually grain-free. Unlike many slow cooker recipes, this one takes only a couple of hours, but it makes an excellent option when you don't have access to your oven or you want an added treat for a brunch or other event. Make sure your bananas are very ripe for best results; the skins should be well spotted with black.

- Coconut oil or unsalted grass-fed butter for greasing
- 2 cups blanched almond flour
- 1 teaspoon baking soda
- 1 teaspoon sea salt
- 1/2 cup chopped and toasted walnuts

- 1/2 cup (1 stick) unsalted grass-fed butter, softened
- 1 cup pure maple syrup
- 2 large eggs
- 2 cups ripe mashed banana
- 3 tablespoons almond milk
- 1 tablespoon pure vanilla extract

Lightly grease the slow cooker crock with coconut oil or butter.

In a large bowl, combine the almond flour, baking soda, salt, and walnuts. Stir well and set aside.

In a separate bowl, using a mixer, beat the butter with the maple syrup. Add the eggs, 1 at a time, beating after each addition. On low speed, beat in the bananas, followed by the almond milk and vanilla. Add the flour mixture and beat until just combined.

Pour the batter into the prepared crock. Cover and cook on high heat for 2 hours. Check doneness by inserting a toothpick. If it's not done, continue cooking on high until a toothpick comes out clean.

Allow the bread to cool, remove from the slow cooker, and slice. Wrap leftover bread in plastic wrap and store at room temperature for up to 3 days.

Serves 8 to 10.

Slow Cooker Almond Bread

This lightly scented almond bread is delicious, and it fits the Paleo plan perfectly. Applesauce makes for a tender and moist bread, while toasted almonds add crunch and flavor. This is the perfect addition to an afternoon tea or a Sunday brunch when served alongside some Paleo-friendly jam. One bite and this is sure to become a favorite.

- Coconut oil or unsalted grass-fed butter for greasing
- 2 cups blanched almond flour
- 1 teaspoon baking soda
- 1 teaspoon sea salt
- 1/2 cup (1 stick) unsalted grass-fed butter, softened

- 1 cup raw honey
- 2 large eggs
- 1 cup unsweetened applesauce
- 3 tablespoon almond milk
- 1 tablespoon pure almond extract
- 1/2 cup sliced almonds, toasted

Lightly grease the slow cooker crock with coconut oil or butter.

In a large bowl, combine the almond flour, baking soda, and salt. Stir well and set aside.

In a separate bowl, using a mixer, beat the butter with the honey. Add the eggs, 1 at a time, beating after each addition. On low speed, beat in the applesauce, followed by the almond milk and extract. Add the flour mixture and beat until just combined.

Pour the batter into the prepared crock. Sprinkle the toasted almonds over the top. Cover and cook on high heat for 2 hours. Check doneness by inserting a toothpick. If it's not done, continue cooking on high until a toothpick comes out clean.

Allow the bread to cool, remove from the slow cooker, and slice. Wrap leftover bread in plastic wrap and store at room temperature for up to 3 days.

Serves 8 to 10.

Toasted Coconut Bread

If you like the taste of coconut, you'll love this lightly sweet bread with toasted coconut on top. This is a wonderful treat to enjoy with a cup of coffee in the morning, and it makes an excellent airy dessert as well. Be sure to use unsweetened shredded coconut for the topping, as sweetened varieties use refined sugar.

- Coconut oil or unsalted grass-fed butter for greasing
- 2 cups blanched almond flour
- 1 tablespoon coconut flour
- 1 teaspoon baking soda
- 1 teaspoon sea salt
- 1/2 cup coconut oil, melted
- 1 cup raw honey
- 2 large eggs
- 1 large ripe banana, mashed
- 3 tablespoons full-fat canned coconut milk
- 1 tablespoon pure vanilla extract
- 1/2 cup unsweetened shredded coconut, toasted

Lightly grease the slow cooker crock with coconut oil or butter.

In a large bowl, combine the almond flour, coconut flour, baking soda, and salt. Stir well and set aside.

In a separate bowl, using a mixer, beat the coconut oil with the honey. Add the eggs, 1 at a time, beating after each addition. On low speed, beat in the banana, followed by the coconut milk and vanilla. Add the flour mixture and beat until just combined.

Pour the batter into the prepared crock. Sprinkle the toasted coconut over the top. Cover and cook on high heat for 2 hours. Check doneness by inserting a toothpick. If it's not done, continue cooking on high until a toothpick comes out clean.

Allow the bread to cool, remove from the slow cooker, and slice. Wrap leftover bread in plastic wrap and store at room temperature for up to 3 days.

Serves 8 to 10.

Slow Cooker Pumpkin Bread

This savory bread is a perfect fall treat, and anyone who tastes it will beg for the recipe. It's best served warm with butter. Feel free to substitute mashed and pureed butternut squash or even sweet potatoes for a twist on this classic bread.

- Coconut oil or unsalted grass-fed butter for greasing
- 2 cups blanched almond flour
- 1 teaspoon baking soda
- 1 teaspoon sea salt
- 2 teaspoons ground cinnamon
- 1/4 teaspoon ground nutmeg
- 1/2 cup (1 stick) unsalted grass-fed butter, softened
- 1 cup pure maple syrup
- 2 large eggs
- 2 cups pureed pumpkin
- 3 tablespoons unsweetened almond milk
- 1 tablespoon pure vanilla extract
- 1/2 cup chopped pecans, toasted (optional)

Lightly grease the slow cooker crock with coconut oil or butter.

In a large bowl, combine the almond flour, baking soda, salt, cinnamon, and nutmeg. Stir well and set aside.

In a separate bowl, using a mixer, beat the butter with the maple syrup and add the eggs, 1 at a time, beating after each addition. On low speed, beat in the pumpkin, followed by the almond milk and vanilla. Add the flour mixture, and beat until batter is just coming together.

Pour the batter into the prepared crock. Sprinkle the toasted pecans over the top, if using. Cover and cook on high heat for 2 hours. Check doneness by inserting a toothpick. If it's not done, continue cooking on high until a toothpick comes out clean.

Allow the bread to cool, remove from the slow cooker, and slice. Wrap leftover bread in plastic wrap and store at room temperature for up to 3 days.

Serves 8 to 10.

Moist and Tender Zucchini Bread

This Paleo version of zucchini bread will rival any traditional recipe when it comes to flavor. Like many quick breads, it retains its moisture for several days after baking, but it is best served warm from the slow cooker. When choosing zucchini, select those on the smaller side, as they tend to be more flavorful and contain more water than the giant ones you often see at farmers' markets and festivals.

- Coconut oil or unsalted grass-fed butter for greasing
- 2 cups blanched almond flour
- 1 tablespoon coconut flour
- 1 teaspoon baking soda
- 1 teaspoon sea salt
- 2 teaspoons ground cinnamon
- 1/2 cup chopped walnuts, toasted
- 1/2 cup coconut oil, melted
- 1 cup raw honey or maple syrup
- 2 large eggs
- 1 cup grated zucchini
- 3 tablespoons almond milk
- 1 tablespoon pure vanilla extract

Lightly grease the slow cooker crock with coconut oil or butter.

In a large bowl, combine the almond flour, coconut flour, baking soda, salt, cinnamon, and walnuts. Stir well and set aside.

In a separate bowl, using a mixer, beat the coconut oil with the honey. Add the eggs, 1 at a time, beating after each addition. On low speed, beat in the zucchini, followed by the almond milk and vanilla. Add the flour mixture and beat until just combined.

Pour the batter into the prepared crock. Cover and cook on high heat for 2 hours. Check doneness by inserting a toothpick. If it's not done, continue cooking on high until a toothpick comes out clean.

Allow the bread to cool, remove from the slow cooker, and slice. Wrap leftover bread in plastic wrap and store at room temperature for up to 3 days.

Serves 8 to 10.

Apple-Cranberry Cobbler

The scent of apple and cinnamon will waft through your house as this cobbler cooks in your slow cooker. The end result is a buttery, bubbly, sweet, and tart dessert that is best served on a chilly fall day. You can use honey for the topping if that's all you have on hand, but maple syrup is definitely recommended.

For the filling:

- Coconut oil or unsalted grass-fed butter for greasing
- 6 large apples, such as Golden Delicious, peeled, cored, and chopped
- 2 cups pure fresh cranberries
- 1 cup raw honey or maple syrup
- 1 tablespoon coconut flour
- 1 teaspoon ground cinnamon
- 1 teaspoon ground cloves
- 1/4 teaspoon ground nutmeg
- 1/4 teaspoon ground ginger

For the topping:

- 1 cup (2 sticks) unsalted grass-fed butter, melted
- 2 cups blanched almond flour
- 1/4 cup pure maple syrup
- 2 large eggs, beaten

Make the filling:

Brush the slow cooker crock with coconut oil or butter.

Add the apples, cranberries, honey, coconut flour, cinnamon, cloves, nutmeg, and ginger to the slow cooker. Stir well to combine.

Make the topping:

In a large bowl, combine the melted butter, almond flour, maple syrup, and eggs. Mix until thoroughly combined.

Spread the topping evenly over the apple mixture. Cover and cook on high heat for about 2 hours. A toothpick inserted into the center of the cobbler should come out completely clean.

Allow the cobbler to cool for 30 minutes, then serve warm. Cover any leftover cobbler and store in the refrigerator for up to 3 days.

Serves 8.

Lemon Poppy Seed Cake

Looking for a light dessert that's still delectable? Look no further than this scrumptious lemon poppy seed cake that is not only Paleo friendly but also made in your slow cooker! Lining the slow cooker crock with parchment paper makes it even better because there's no cleanup. How can you beat that?

- 2 1/2 cups blanched almond flour
- 1 tablespoon baking soda
- 1/2 teaspoon sea salt
- 1/2 cup (1 stick) unsalted grass-fed butter, softened
- 1 cup raw honey
- 2 large eggs
- 1 teaspoon pure vanilla extract
- Zest of 1 lemon
- 1 tablespoon poppy seeds

In a medium bowl, combine the almond flour, baking soda, and salt. Set aside.

In a large bowl, using a mixer, beat the butter with the honey until smooth. Beat in the eggs, 1 at time, and mix until creamy. Add the vanilla and lemon zest and beat on low until smooth. Add the flour mixture and beat until smooth. Fold in the poppy seeds.

Lay a large piece of parchment paper in the slow cooker crock, making sure there is plenty overhanging the edges. Pour in the cake batter.

Cover and cook over low heat for about 2 hours, or until a toothpick inserted in the center comes out clean. The edges of the cake should be browned and starting to pull away from the sides.

Allow the cake to cool for 20 minutes in the slow cooker, then lift it out by pulling up on the sides of the parchment. Cut the cake into squares and serve warm. Wrap leftover cake in plastic wrap and store at room temperature for up to 3 days.

Serves 8 to 10.

Maple-Baked Apples

Tart dried cherries and crunchy walnuts enhance maple-scented apples in this slow cooker dessert that's a breeze to put together. These apples make an impressive dinner party treat and are perfect for when you're lacking oven space. Start them during dinner, and by the time you've cleaned up and relaxed for a few minutes, dessert is ready with little effort on your part. Your guests will never know that these are actually Paleo friendly. Granny Smith apples are an excellent choice here; they are firm and hold up well, plus they aren't loaded with sugar like some varieties. For an interesting variation to this recipe, you can also try using pears.

- 4 medium apples, cored
- 1/4 cup chopped walnuts
- 1/4 cup dried cherries
- 1 teaspoon ground cinnamon
- 1/2 cup pure maple syrup
- 1/2 cup apple cider

Arrange the apples in the slow cooker.

In a small bowl, combine the walnuts, cherries, and cinnamon. Mix well, then divide the mixture evenly between the apples, filling the cored centers. Drizzle the maple syrup over the apples and pour the apple cider into the slow cooker.

Cover and cook on low heat for about 2 hours. Remove the lid and allow the apples to cool for about 10 minutes before serving.

Place the apples on plates and drizzle the cooking liquid over the top. Leftover apples can be stored in an airtight container in the refrigerator for up to 3 days.

Serves 4.

Slow Cooker Chocolate Cake

The slow cooker is a great addition to the Paleo diet, but you can do more than braise meats and turn out mouthwatering stews. This chocolate cake recipe proves that. This moist chocolate cake is even better than many traditional recipes you'll find. It's more rich than sweet, but feel free to add a bit more honey if you like sweeter desserts.

- Coconut oil or unsalted grass-fed butter for greasing
- 2 cups blanched almond flour
- 3/4 cup unsweetened cocoa powder
- 2 teaspoons baking soda
- 1 teaspoon sea salt
- 1 cup raw honey
- 1 large egg
- 1 cup almond milk
- 1/2 cup coconut oil
- 1 tablespoon pure vanilla extract
- 1 cup boiling water

Brush the slow cooker crock with coconut oil or butter.

In a large bowl, combine the almond flour, cocoa powder, baking soda, and salt. Stir well.

In a separate bowl, beat the honey, egg, almond milk, coconut oil, and vanilla together with a mixer. Add to the flour mixture. Pour in the boiling water and stir well to combine.

Pour the batter into the slow cooker, cover, and cook on low heat for about 3 hours. The cake is done when the top is dry and the edges are starting to pull away from the sides.

Uncover and allow the cake to cool for about 30 minutes before serving. Store leftover cake loosely covered at room temperature until ready to serve. It will keep well in the refrigerator for up to 1 week in an airtight container.

Serves 8.

Slow Cooker Paleo Brownies

Looking for a rich and chocolaty dessert that's made in your slow cooker? How about one that is also gluten-free and Paleo friendly? If that's what you're looking for, you've hit the jackpot with these brownies. Chocolate cravings will be satisfied with one bite of these sinfully delicious and chewy delights. Serve them at your next party; your guests won't believe they are actually suitable for a diet.

- 1 1/2 cups blanched almond flour
- 1/2 cup unsweetened cocoa powder
- 1 teaspoon baking soda
- 1/2 teaspoon sea salt
- 1/2 cup (1 stick) unsalted grass-fed butter, melted
- 1 cup raw honey
- 2 large eggs, beaten

Line the slow cooker crock with aluminum foil.

In a small bowl, combine the almond flour, cocoa powder, baking soda, and salt.

In a medium bowl, combine the melted butter and honey. Add the eggs and whisk until well combined. Add the flour mixture and stir until well blended.

Pour the batter into the prepared crock. Cover and cook on low heat for about 3 hours. Uncover and cook for 30 more minutes.

Allow the brownies to cool completely before removing the foil, slicing, and serving. Store any leftover brownies in an airtight container for up to 3 days.

Serves 12.

SECTION TWO

Living Paleo and Gluten-Free

WHAT IS THE PALEO DIET?

The Paleo diet has also been called the Stone Age diet, a name derived from the book *The Stone Age Diet,* published in 1975 by gastroenterologist Walter Voegtlin. Voegtlin's book was based on years of studying his patients on a diet composed largely of meats and small quantities of carbohydrates from vegetables, nuts, and seeds. He reported that many of his patients, who suffered from problems such as Crohn's Disease and irritable bowel syndrome, showed marked improvement while on the diet (Voegtlin 1975).

Unfortunately, the mid-seventies were a time when everyone was certain that saturated fats were to be avoided at all costs and fruits and grains were two of the food groups that should be eaten in abundance.

It wasn't until ten years later, when Boyd Eaton and Melvin Konner published their research in the *New England Journal of Medicine,* that the medical community and a few members of the public began to seriously consider the merits of the Stone Age diet. This research led to the publishing of *The Paleolithic Prescription: A Program of Diet and Exercise and a Design for Living,* with Marjorie Shostak. The book has served as the foundation for today's version of the Paleo diet.

The Paleolithic Prescription explained that although mankind's history can be traced back at least 2.5 million years, man didn't start growing and eating grains until about ten thousand years ago. The book also pointed out that when people started heavily eating processed foods and grain-based products in the twentieth century, obesity, heart disease, and a host of other problems began to increase (Eaton, Shostak, and Konner 1988).

The decision to go on the Paleo diet basically boils down to one question: Do you think you should eat the way you were designed to eat or the way that you've become accustomed to eating?

The Basics of the Paleo Diet

Although there are several versions of the Paleo diet, they all are based on the same basic principle: eating a diet more like that of our Paleo ancestors, which would exclude processed foods, grains, legumes, dairy, refined sugars, and most alcohol.

Many people were concerned that a diet that was meat-centric had to be unhealthful for the heart and arteries, but several studies have shown that the Paleo guideline of eating grass-fed organic meats is very healthful indeed.

Did You Know? *A 2009 research study conducted by Clemson University and the USDA showed that, compared to feedlot meats, grass-fed meats are higher in antioxidants, vitamins, and minerals; lower in the saturated fats associated with heart disease; lower in total fat; and higher in CLA, which is thought to fight some cancers. It also has a higher amount of omega-3 fatty acids and a healthier ratio of omega-3 to omega-6 fats (Duckett et al. 2009).*

Aside from focusing on a meat-centric diet, the Paleo diet also omits all grains and legumes, as these foods were not eaten by humans until just ten thousand years ago. The scientific community that has studied the Paleolithic era diet maintains (and several studies have shown) that ten thousand years isn't nearly enough time for our genes to have modified to the degree that our bodies can easily digest or benefit from grains and legumes.

Because of obvious health concerns that aren't exclusive to the Paleo diet, alcohol, refined sugars, and dairy are also excluded from the diet.

The Paleo diet isn't by any means sparse. Calorie counting is generally frowned upon, and followers are invited to eat as much as they want of most meats, vegetables, fruits, nuts, seeds, and healthful oils, such as coconut, olive, walnut, and palm oil.

Fans of the Paleo diet often remark on the amount of food they're able to eat, the satisfaction they feel, and how much they appreciate the freedom from counting calories, carb grams, and other data throughout the day.

The Benefits of the Paleo Diet

There are several very important health benefits to eating according to the Paleo diet.

As previously discussed, grass-fed meats and organic, free-range poultry are significantly higher in heart-healthful fats and lower in those fats that are connected to heart disease, arterial disease, and stroke.

The absence of processed foods such as fast foods, packaged snacks, deep-fried treats, and sugary desserts and sodas means that most people take in far fewer calories than on a typical Western diet, which helps them lose weight and keep it off. This makes the diet an excellent one for combating obesity.

The same can be said of the Paleo diet's positive impact on type 2 diabetes and metabolic syndrome. Many studies have shown that the diet's lack of sugar, processed flours, and alcohol can be of great benefit to those with either disease. A study by Lund University found that men with these conditions who followed the Paleo diet for three months showed an improvement in their glucose tolerance by an average of 26 percent (Jönsson et al. 2009).

The Paleo diet is also naturally gluten-free, so it's a healthful and satisfying diet for those who have celiac disease or gluten sensitivity. It's also a safe diet for those with a wheat allergy, as all wheat products are off-limits.

Did You Know? *The consumption of grains, dairy products, and legumes is being blamed more and more for the increase in immune disorders and symptoms of immunity imbalances. Many studies support this theory. In 1998, Dr. Jean Seignalet conducted a study of several hundred patients with various immune disorders who were put on a Paleo diet. Every one of the lupus patients showed at least a 50 percent improvement in their symptoms, as did 97 percent of patients with fibromyalgia and multiple sclerosis (Seignalet 2001).*

Many people report significant weight loss, increased energy, and a greater sense of satiety on the Paleo diet than on other diets. Coupled with the benefits to heart health, type 2 diabetes and metabolic syndrome, and immune disorders, it's not hard to understand why so many people are such strong supporters of the Paleo way of eating.

WHAT IS GLUTEN-FREE?

Gluten-free eating has become incredibly popular worldwide in the last decade. The prevalence of celiac disease, gluten sensitivity, and wheat allergies has meant that more and more people are switching to a gluten-free diet.

The Paleo diet is naturally gluten-free, as it excludes all cereal grains, including wheat, oats, and barley. When the lack of gluten and its unwanted and unhealthful side effects is paired with the other health benefits of the Paleo diet, it just makes good sense for those with gluten issues.

This chapter explains the differences between celiac disease, gluten sensitivity, and wheat allergy; gives you an understanding of what it's like to go without gluten and grain products; and lets you know about all of the benefits you'll reap from following the Paleo diet.

The Basics of Gluten-Free

Many people unfamiliar with a gluten-free diet believe that it means having to give up every kind of bread, cracker, muffin, cake, cookie, and other baked good. Happily, this couldn't be further from the truth.

Although flours made from wheat, rye, barley, oats, and some other cereal grains are most commonly used in making breads and other baked goods, there are a great variety of other flours from which to choose.

People on the Paleo diet successfully make pancakes, quick breads, savory breads, muffins, cookies, and all kinds of other yummy foods with nut meals such as hazelnut flour, walnut flour, coconut flour, and almond flour. Although yeast is not used in Paleo baking, arrowroot powder, baking soda, and baking powder are all allowed and used with wonderful results.

Many studies have shown that after just a couple of weeks on a gluten-free diet, followers show remarkable improvement with gluten-related symptoms such as bloating, gas, loose bowels, inflammation, and fatigue. It's nice to know that benefiting from a gluten-free diet doesn't have to mean living without dinner rolls and blueberry muffins.

A true gluten-free diet that is prescribed for those diagnosed with celiac disease excludes not just grain products, but also some types of vitamins, condiments, beverages, and other products that are made using gluten as a filler or stabilizer. Unless you are diagnosed with celiac or a serious gluten sensitivity, you don't need to go to such extremes. However, you'll likely see many other benefits from avoiding gluten when you take up the Paleo diet.

Did You Know? *If you suspect that you may have celiac disease, it's very important that you don't go on a gluten-free diet before being tested. According to Dr. Stefano Guandalini, founder of The University of Chicago Celiac Disease Center, just a few weeks without gluten can skew the test results for celiac, as they're based on the presence of antibodies (Hill et al. 2005).*

The Benefits of Gluten-Free

Even if you have not been diagnosed with celiac disease or don't have sensitivity to gluten, you can benefit greatly from going on a gluten-free diet such as the Paleo diet.

In the typical Western diet, so many of the day's calories come from breads, baked goods, cereals, and foods processed or made with refined flours. Going on a gluten-free diet means that you automatically eliminate many unhealthful calories from your diet as well as those heavily processed ingredients.

Many people on a gluten-free diet lose at least some weight once they go gluten-free, although you don't have to lose weight if you don't need to. If you see that you're dropping pounds you'd prefer to keep, simply eat more of the foods you're allowed to enjoy.

Even people without celiac or a gluten sensitivity report less bloating, gas, irregularity, inflammation, fatigue, and other symptoms associated with gluten-containing foods.

If you're worried about getting enough carbohydrates, don't be. You'll get plenty of carbs through vegetables, fruits, nuts, and seeds. Admittedly, you'll be eating fewer carbs than the typical American, and you may feel some fatigue or lethargy in the first couple of weeks as a result. However, once your body adjusts to the new carb levels, it will adapt by using proteins for energy more efficiently. One of the most common remarks about the Paleo diet is that people experience a wonderful increase in their energy levels after the first few weeks.

You don't have to suffer from celiac disease or gluten sensitivity to see the benefits of cutting gluten from your diet.

THE BEAUTY OF PALEO SLOW COOKING

S low cooking has a bit of an image problem. People unfamiliar with slow cooking tend to think that it's for people who don't like to cook or don't know how, that it results in mushy or dried-out food, or that it's only good for stews and pot roast.

Preparing food in a slow cooker is actually not much different from slow cooking in a Dutch oven on the stovetop or in the oven. It renders even the toughest meats tender and moist, and it can be used for much more than stews, including breads, breakfasts, roasts, chowders, sides, and even desserts.

The beauty of using the slow cooker method on the Paleo diet is that it saves you time and makes even the most economical meats flavorful and delicious. Whether you're short on time or not, slow cooking is a great way to have dinner ready and waiting when you walk in the door, freeing you up to do all of those other things that make your life richer.

The Basics of Slow Cooking

This cookbook is a collection of recipes to be prepared using one of the many slow cookers available on the market.

You can buy slow cookers with volume capacities ranging from three quarts to twelve quarts, and in all price ranges. The recipes in this book were written for a six-quart model, which is very common and easy to find at any big-box store for as little as twenty dollars.

Many slow cookers come with automatic timers and shutoffs, but you don't need any bells and whistles to enjoy using your slow cooker. Most recipes take six to eight hours, allowing you to turn the slow cooker on before you leave for work without worrying about the food becoming overcooked.

In general, you can extend the cooking time if you need to by using the low heat setting when the recipe calls for high heat. For meat dishes, it's not recommended that you do the reverse, however, as this could result in the meat being tough.

Using the slow cooker locks in all the flavors of your ingredients; nothing is lost through evaporation as it would be with many other cooking methods. This also preserves the vitamin content of your foods.

Slow cookers save you time not just with cooking but with cleanup as well. One-pot meals are a great way to cut down on the number of dishes that need to be washed after dinner. Most slow cookers have removable stoneware inserts that you can lift out of the slow cooker and wash very easily. You can also buy slow cooker liners in the food storage aisle at the supermarket if you'd like to avoid washing up altogether.

Once you get the hang of using a slow cooker and have some idea of how certain ingredients fare, you'll find that it'll be quite easy for you to convert your own favorite Paleo recipes to the slow cooker.

Did You Know? *Some newer models of slow cookers are even more versatile. There are versions on the market that allow you to use the crock insert either as part of the slow cooker or directly in the oven. You can even brown the meat in the insert right on the stovetop before transferring it into the heating base. These models definitely earn their storage space.*

Tips for Slow Cooking

- If you have a slow cooker that is smaller than six quarts, try halving the recipe or increasing the cook time by about 20 percent.

- Try not to remove the cover of your slow cooker during cooking. The slow cooker loses a great deal of heat when the lid is removed and this can result in uneven cooking. If you can't resist peeking, you'll need to increase the cooking time by as much as 30 minutes every time you lift that lid.

- One hour on high heat equals approximately two hours on low heat. If you need to let your slow cooker cook longer or if you'd like the meal done sooner, that conversion is generally safe. Use caution when cooking large, tougher cuts of meat, as switching from low to high heat may mean that it turns out less tender.

- Browning meat before putting it into the slow cooker seals in the juices and reduces some of the fat. It's not necessary for all meats, but don't skip this step if it's included in the recipe.

- Even though the volume of liquid called for in a recipe may seem inadequate when compared to traditional cooking methods, since none of it is lost to evaporation, what you put in is generally what you end up with.

- Harder vegetables take longer to cook in the slow cooker than many meats. Put root vegetables on the bottom of the slow cooker and meats on top.

- Never put the slow cooker in water. Pull out the stoneware insert for easy cleaning. Also, be sure to let the insert cool for some time before putting it in cool water, as it could crack or warp over time.

Did You Know? *High cooking temperatures and steam can account for the loss of as much as 80 percent of the vitamin content of your food. Using the slow cooker allows you to preserve the vitamins and minerals in your food because it cooks at a slow, low temperature in a sealed vessel.*

Paleo Slow Cooking

Slow cooking and the Paleo diet were meant to be together.

The focus on meats and fresh vegetables means that the Paleo diet can sometimes be cooking-intensive, at least when it comes to time. Many people on the Paleo diet have busy schedules that don't leave much time or energy for cooking at the end of a hard day.

Using the slow cooker for preparing your Paleo meals means that a few minutes of prep is all you need to get dinner going before you leave for work. When you get home, dinner is ready and waiting for you. You can even do most of the preparation for your dinner the night before when you may have a bit more time or while you're preparing another meal. With most recipes, you can get everything prepped and into the crock insert, store it in the refrigerator overnight, and place the insert into the heating base in the morning.

Slow cooking also takes some of the pressure out of eating Paleo on a budget. The focus on grass-fed and organic foods means that grocery items can be more expensive to buy. This can end up causing you to get stuck eating foods you don't particularly care for simply because they're cheap, or buying a lower-quality product because funds are tight.

Slow cooking allows you to take the less expensive cuts of meat and turn them into a tender, flavorful meal that only low, slow cooking can produce. This frees up some of your budget for purchasing other quality ingredients.

The Paleo diet lends itself very well to soups and stews; you'll find hundreds of recipes in cookbooks and online. The slow cooker is a great way to prepare them, but they aren't your only option for delicious slow-cooked meals. The slow cooker is also excellent for roasts, breads, vegetables, and even desserts.

The timesaving features and economy of using a slow cooker blend beautifully with the health goals and busy lifestyles of those on the Paleo diet.

CONCLUSION

You now have a great head start on your Paleo and gluten-free slow-cooking adventure. But don't stop with these recipes; convert your old family favorites to the slow cooker and have fun experimenting with other recipes from all over the world.

The Paleo diet is full of a wonderful array of foods, and there are at least a dozen ways to prepare each one of them in the slow cooker.

With a slow cooker and the abundant choices available on the Paleo diet, there's no reason to get stuck in a food rut or to approach the dinner table with resignation. Get creative, experiment with unfamiliar ingredients or seasonings, and invest some time checking out cuisines that you may not have tried before.

Going Paleo is all about looking great, feeling wonderful, and getting the most out of your life. Paleo slow cooking helps you accomplish all three.

REFERENCES

Duckett, S. K., J. P. S. Neel, J. P. Fontenot, and W. M. Clapham. 2009. "Effects of Winter Stocker Growth Rate and Finishing System on: III Tissue Proximate, Fatty Acid, Vitamin and Cholesterol Content." *Journal of Animal Science* 87 (September): 2,961 70. doi: 10.2527/jas.2009-1850.

Eaton, S. Boyd, and Marvin Konner. 1985. "Paleolithic Nutrition: A Consideration of Its Nature and Current Implications." *The New England Journal of Medicine* 312 (5): 283–89.

Eaton, S. Boyd, Marjorie Shostak, and Marvin Konner. 1988. *The Paleolithic Prescription: A Programme of Diet and Exercise and a Design for Living.* New York: Harper & Row.

Hill, Ivor D., Martha H. Dirks, Gregoy S. Liptak, Richard B. Colletti, Alessio Fasano, Stefano Guandalini, Edward J. Hoffenberg, Karoly Horvath, Joseph A. Murray, Mitchell Pivor, and Ernest G. Seidman. 2005. North American Society for Pediatric Gastroenterology, Hepatology and Nutrition. "Guideline for the Diagnosis and Treatment of Celiac Disease in Children: Recommendations of the North American Society for Pediatric Gastroenterology, Hepatology and Nutrition." *Journal of Pediatric Gastroenterology and Nutrition* 40 (1): 17–18.

Jönsson, Tommy, Yvonne Granfeldt, Bo Ahrén, Ulla-Carin Branell, Gunvor Pålsson, Anita Hansson, Margareta Söderström, and Staffan Lindeberg. 2009. "Beneficial Effects of a Paleolithic Diet on Cardiovascular Risk Factors in Type 2 Diabetes: A Randomized Crossover Study." *Cardiovascular Diabetology* 8: 35. doi: 10.1186/1475-2840-8-35.

Seignalet, Jean. 2001. *L'Alimentation ou la troisième médecine*, 3rd ed. Paris, FR: F. X. de Guibert.

Voegtlin, Walter L. 1975. *The Stone Age Diet: Based on In-Depth Studies of Human Ecology and the Diet of Man*. New York: Vantage Press.

CPSIA information can be obtained at www.ICGtesting.com
Printed in the USA
LVOW05s0125090114

368700LV00002B/298/P